Truly Healthy Now

A Guide to Attaining
Enlightenment
in Health and Fitness

by

David Léasure

Important Note To Readers:

This book is not intended to replace the advice of your healthcare professional or physician. You should consult a healthcare professional before adopting any nutrition or exercise advice in this program or in any new exercise program you undertake, especially if you are new to exercise or have any existing health problems.

For my dad.

CONTENTS

INTRODUCTION

When I was younger I wanted to look like Rocky. It wasn't until my older brother started working out that I did too. Originally I refused, but somehow I got into it. Fast forward a few years and I joined the Navy right after high school. It was the first time in my life I had a real paycheck, and I spent it on an online bodybuilding course. Over the next few months I devoted myself body, mind, and soul to that program. I exercised like crazy, ate what I was told to eat, and took all of the exercise supplements I was told to take. I felt great and was on top of the world. Or so I thought.

Deployment hit me like a sack of rocks. Everything I had worked for— everything—went out the porthole (some sailor humor). I went from normal working hours to over fifteen. I went from two open gyms to two tiny gyms. I went from precision-timing my supplement intake to not even having enough room to store them! I thought everything was ruined.

Serendipity is a funny thing, and it just so happened that a gentleman I worked with was also into fitness. But his was eccentric. Instead of worshiping muscle heads, he was into calisthenics, which if you're familiar, is the use of your body weight to exercise. He lent me two books that completely changed my life: *Convict Conditioning 2* by, Paul "Coach" Wade, and *Solitary Fitness* by, Charles Bronson (the infamous UK inmate). I devoured these books, but the big reason they meant so much to me was because they felt relatable. I did not feel so alone anymore on my floating fortress. These men did the best they could with little to no resources. They lacked the one thing you should lack in an exercise toolkit: excuses.

Fast-forward to shore, and I'm still struggling which route to take. You would think it'd be an easy decision now that I saw the light, but I was married to the gym, and getting off of lifting for aesthetic reasons was like getting off a deeply addicting drug. Should I continue exercising bare-bones, calisthenics, eating only what was provided me? Or should I go back to my bodybuilding and supplement routine? The problem was, I had seen reality, and my ego was deeply shattered. The illusion behind the curtain was revealed. There was no going back.

Over the course of the next few years, I devoted myself to continuously shaving my ego, the way a farmer might whittle down a stick. Not working out just to look better, but to be better. To be healthy, and to find out what fitness really was.

This book isn't strictly about calisthenics, or why weights are bad. It's just about finding a deeper meaning to your fitness, beyond the ego.

Chapter Zero

Big Questions

What are we doing here? Why have we let ourselves go? When I received my first paycheck, one of the things I immediately did was invest in an online exercise program. I did pretty well, too. I worked out hard and thought I had finally found what I had been looking for: a lean, muscular body. But I soon realized that this wasn't actually healthy. I looked the part but was I? I am lazy by nature. Not lazy in the sense that I like to lay on the couch all day and eat potato chips, but in the sense that to get myself to do anything, I have to understand why. I began scraping the bottom of the barrel, wondering what in the world I was exercising for anymore. One day I woke up physically (and mentally) exhausted. As I lay in my bed, supposed to be getting up to go to the gym, I started asking myself some questions. Some *big* questions.

Why am I doing this?

Am I really getting anything out of this anymore?

If this is making me a better person, how so?

I looked bigger, great! But was that the only reason, to look better in front of other people? Well, yeah! What other reason could there be? I just didn't feel the pizazz anymore—the desire to train. I had lost the fire in me that had kept me going for so long.

Why am I exercising?

I was only exercising to look better, that was it. Now that may sound like an admirable thing because that's what we're all striving for, right? But it just wasn't enough anymore. And it certainly wasn't enough to get me out of bed in the early hours of the morning. I decided then and there that my training was no longer going to simply be about getting bigger or looking better. It was going to be about being healthy and having a functional body.

Something major had happened to me, I had had a shift in perspective.

This is where most of us fail. Not only on our fitness journeys but most importantly, in our health. But what is it that crumbles away and makes us give up? Why do we never go the distance? I'd wager it's our foundations, or lack thereof. When a weak foundation falls away, you have to have the courage to build a new, stronger one. We do things for all of the wrong reasons: we're told to eat better, to look better, to *be* better. But what is *better*? When something isn't working, we usually try harder or go faster, when what we *really* need to be doing is to let go and reevaluate.

"Everyone who hears these words and does them will be like the wise man who built his house on the rock. And the rain fell, and the floods came, and the winds blew and beat on the house, but it did not fall, because it had been founded on the rock." Matthew 7:24

Is my ego getting the better of me?

Not everyone you see who looks great with their shirt off is actually healthy. In all reality, a lot of them are probably doing something harmful to their bodies—whether wittingly or unwittingly—to look the way they do. You don't have to have two percent body fat or softball-sized biceps in order to be considered healthy.

I am an ectomorph by nature. That means I am skinny and have a hard time gaining muscle. When I started my amateur bodybuilding routine, my goal was to gain lots of muscle weight. Healthy? But this is healthy, right? Well I suppose if you think eating a whole lot one week, then starving yourself the next, thus ruining your metabolism is, then yes. I was young and naïve, so this was what I thought being healthy was: how I looked.

And it was good for a while, I got a lot of praise:

"Hey, looking swole!"

"Look out, Schwarzenegger coming through!"

It was great and I loved what people were saying. But the starving myself, overeating, and spending three hours in the gym each day, six days a week just wasn't working anymore. In the end, I forgot why I was even working out in the first place. To please others? So that people wouldn't poke fun at my size?

This was something I had to meditate on for a long time before coming to a conclusion. I decided that I wouldn't care anymore about what people thought of how I looked. What was important was how healthy I was and how physically I felt.

CHAPTER ONE

ENVYING OTHERS

We've all been there before: in the gym, at the park, in the woods. We've psyched ourselves to go work out. We're not entirely sure of EVERYTHING we're doing, but we're trying, and that's the important thing. Our faces turn red because we feel everyone might be staring at us. After a few minutes we catch a glimpse of ourselves in the mirror: *well, that's a little disappointing.* Then we see him or her, that person who looks amazing in their workout clothes. It's in that moment everything falls apart:

"Why even bother?"

"What's the point?"

"I'll never look like that."

And just like that we quit before we really even started.

Focus on YOU.

When you exercise you need to develop a laser-sharp focus, a focus that dissolves everything around you. You have only one thing to think about: your workout. We all get nervous. We worry what others will think about us, from our hair to our shoes. But the reality is, people in the gym are there to work on *themselves*. They're too busy to worry about you.

Fitness is a Journey

Being healthy is not a place you get to, it's a place of being. You'll have good days and you'll have bad days, but every day in some way, you are bettering yourself. It can be difficult because as human beings we get jealous easily. We look at someone with the body we want and are envious. We look at a magazine cover and are then embarrassed by our own bodies. But there is no shame in bettering yourself, in anything you do. Whether they're Olympic Gold Medalists or Heavy-Weight Champions, everyone has to start out somewhere. And even when they get to the "top" they still train, perhaps not competitively, but to better themselves. I don't care if you've never worked out a day in your life or since you were in diapers, there's always a way to better yourself. And you can do it starting right now.

Comparing Yourself to Others

Any magazine you pick up is going to make you feel like crap: BIGGER ARMS, smaller thighs, diets out the eardrum. These magazines are great until they start contradicting themselves: Don't do that, do this! Discover the NEW way to burn body fat and sculpt OLYMPIAN ABS. If you pick up this garbage, your head is going to spin and you'll have wasted precious brain cells and time from your life. These are gimmicks, and no matter what they say, they don't care about you, they just want your attention.

If you are going to start this journey, you must understand something very clearly: If you continue to compare your body to others you will only get depressed, unmotivated, and ultimately quit. When you focus on health instead, and your own progress, you'll find that you don't want or *need* to compare yourself to others. You won't view them with envy, but see them simply as other people on the same journey as you.

Rivers shape bedrock

Let go and flow with the water. From the outside, it looks like the water isn't doing much, just flowing along. But the river *exists* because the water is constantly pushing against and shaping the rock beneath it. Start from where you are and go from there. Not with the idea that you want to change yourself, but with the idea that you want to move forward. You will get to where you need to be and make a bigger impact on your body and health than you ever imagined.

CHAPTER TWO

UNMOORING THE BOAT

There are many distractions when it comes to health and fitness. We get so wrapped up in our own egos and what other people think that we don't even bother exercising correctly anymore. If you could eliminate these distractions, you could see the goal clearer in your mind. Take away the vanity, the jealousy, and the ego and you're left with only yourself. Who are you when all the gimmicks are taken away?

> *"We burn the fat off our souls."*
> -Ernest Hemmingway

Tossing out the scale

One of the worst things you can do to yourself on your health journey is to worry about numbers on a scale. Why is this? Aren't scales supposed to help keep us on track? Well, yes and no. Scales are good for one thing: telling you numbers, that's it. But we spend so much time worrying about how much we weigh that we miss the point. What a waste of time it is to worry about something so fickle and ultimately miss the big picture. People will overeat and undereat, and in severe cases even resort to bulimia or anorexia. This is a problem that all starts in your mind, thinking there's something wrong with how you look or who you are.

What? No scale! Come on honey, this guy's a crackpot. Let's go to the checkout aisle, I thought I saw an interesting new edition of "Male Ego!"

Your health is more important than numbers on a scale. But people will do whatever it takes to weigh less, even if it means doing something harmful to their body. I was so embarrassed of my weight when I was younger. No matter what I did that darn number on the scale would never change. And then something happened, I took a bodybuilding course. My physicality changed, but the number on the scale didn't. Then something else happened, I got off the bodybuilding course and trained advanced calisthenics. Again, my physicality changed but the number on the scale didn't. Why not? I believe because my body was balancing itself out. But do you think I cared about this? All I wanted was that number to rise! The number on a scale is so insignificant but we give it so much power. People are more concerned about how much they weigh than their actual health. If someone was told they could cut out thirty pounds by increasing their cholesterol, they'd probably do it. The number on your scale is the last thing that's important. The first thing is your health. And if your body truly needs to lose weight, or gain it, it will. But as an after effect to exercise. Health goes beyond numbers.

I'm not trying to belittle the scale here, rather our use of it. When people see the numbers aren't tipping in their favor, they quit. I understand some of us may have to lose weight for medical reasons, but it's not something to obsess over. That will just make things worse. If you need to watch your weight, check every few weeks, but not every day.

> *"You must unlearn what you have learned."*
> -Yoda

Accepting yourself

I always hear people say,

"If only I was thinner!"

"If only I was taller!"

"Then I would be happy! Then I would be content!"

Only when you accept who you are can you begin to make adjustments. Until you appreciate and acknowledge who you are *right now*, in this moment, you won't be able to get any real work done. You're not chasing an image or a persona. You're taking responsibility for yourself and treating yourself with respect. If you don't, when you do hit that ideal weight you've been striving for, you'll only find something else to criticize about yourself.

Less mirror, please

There's nothing more degrading to yourself than spending copious amounts of time looking at yourself in the mirror, even if you have the greatest body in the world. You look at something too often or too long, and your mind WILL find something to complain about it.

- *You're too fat.*

- *You're too skinny.*

- *Your muscles look like dried raisins.*

- *You've got TOO MUCH "junk in the trunk."*

The list goes on and on. You're making more progress than you think. But because you are the judge and jury, even when other people compliment you, you think to yourself, "Yes, but this is wrong with me and I still have to work on *that*."

I came to the mirror conclusion some years ago and it is by far one of the best things I could tell someone about exercising or loving their body. It's amazing how much we drive ourselves crazy by constantly analyzing and scrutinizing every tiny detail about ourselves. Don't get me wrong, it's good to have constructive criticism—and people will give you plenty of that— but constantly looking at your body in the mirror and degrading yourself will do you no good. A glance, a look over. That's fine. But flopping the arms around or constantly looking at the skinny legs will depress you and ultimately make you quit. Learn to love your body because I'll tell you right now, not all bodies are the same. The most successful athletes understand that and work to balance their strengths and weaknesses.

And remember, not all mirrors are created equal. Some make you look fat, some make you look skinny. And then there's the lighting. The factors that play into your "appearance" are endless.

Bite-size

I see these exercise bundles, they've got like, twenty DVDs, ten books, seven PDFs, twelve MP3s. Stop! Stop! Stop! There's a reason why they want you to buy the whole thing in one go instead of one at a time. They know that most people are only going to get through the first few DVDs and then quit. Fortunately for the company, they already got their money. But why do people quit? Because there's so much information that it becomes overwhelming! Instead of taking everything one at a time, they start to panic and think to themselves, "Oh God, I'm only on DVD one. There are twenty DVDs!" All of a sudden the work becomes longer, the kids become louder, the spouse becomes more annoying, and before you know it, "I quit! That's it, I'm done. I quit!" Or worse, the exercise just slips quietly into the background. One day turns into three. One week turns into four, and before you know it, it's two months later and you haven't exercised at all.

Many of us psych ourselves to do things rather than take a minute to understand why we're doing them in the first place. We get caught up in the glamor, the loud infomercial, the pretty looking product and think, *I want that*. Because all it takes is just a little push, the *order now before it's too late* forces us to pick up the phone. One week later it arrives and we're looking at a butt load of stuff. We're looking at a butt load of work.

If you try to see your entire fitness journey in one panorama, you won't make it through. Take things one day at a time, one workout at a time, one meal at a time.

Inch by inch, life is a cinch. Mile by mile, life is a trial. Exercise and fitness is a journey, and the journey of a thousand miles begins with the first step. Focus on that first step and then the next, and then the next. Keep walking and before you know it you'll be like The Winter Warlock who walked right out the door.[1]

An ever-changing body

The body can be pretty weird sometimes. In the beginning of the day you are taller, at the end of the day you are shorter.[2] And in the morning you carry less weight because you haven't had anything to eat or drink for hours.[3] Some people love this, especially those who are trying to lose weight. But on the other hand, for us smaller guys trying to GAIN weight, it can be a real nightmare. Imagine a guy who works out for three hours and eats a ton of food throughout the day because he's trying to put on some weight. Before he goes to bed, he checks himself in the mirror. *Not too bad*, he thinks. *It's all uphill from here.* Then he wakes up, looks in the mirror and is mortified to see who is staring back at him: Jack Skellington! *Where's all that hard work I put in? I looked great last night! What happened?* He doesn't understand that his body is always changing. It's a never-ending game of cat and mouse.

Now let's look at someone trying to lose weight. After eating just a small meal, they're bloated. They see their gut sticking out and are heartbroken. *I just ate a light meal, what happened?* But that's just it, they're only bloated. They'll come down from it soon enough. There is no singular *body* that exists. You are a constantly changing, always fluctuating mass of epic proportions.

Chapter Three

Different Body Types

We're constantly bombarded with what the "perfect body" should look like. It's fed to us on a daily basis in magazines, social media, and movies. Guys are supposed to be tall with broad shoulders, and girls are supposed to be thin with a nice chest and butt, Botticelli's Venus. But bodies are not created equal, they come in all shapes and sizes. Each with its own advantages and disadvantages.

These are the three basic body types:

- Ectomorph
- Endomorph
- Mesomorph

Ectomorph

These body types are generally quite skinny. Ectomorphs have a very high metabolism and so are able to take in much more calories than the average person and gain little to no weight in the process. I am an ectomorph and so I was always told that I had to eat more than I was used to in order to gain weight. As I got older though, I realized that the people who were telling me this didn't know or care who I was, so I dropped it. I don't believe in gluttony or over-eating; it's a waste of food someone else could have. Instead I eat until I've had my fill and leave it at that.

Endomorph

This body type gains weight more easily than the others. Now, there is a difference between being a naturally bigger person and being obese. America has its obesity problem, I don't need to tell you that. But this body type may be more susceptible to it. In America specifically, we seem to reside on either one of two sides on a vast spectrum. Either we're very fit and health-conscious, or we're obese and unhealthy. It's okay to be big! If you're big, you're big! *But be healthy*. Don't for one second think there's something wrong with you because you're a naturally bigger person. I'm not trying to feed you sugar pills because here's some vinegar: you may be obese. You may be unhealthy. But it all comes down to your lifestyle. What do you eat? How much do you eat? Do you exercise? If you eat well and maintain a healthy lifestyle, chances are you're just big. But if you don't take care of your body, it doesn't matter even if you are a mesomorph (see below). The point I'm trying to make is that it's not about how you look, or what you've been impressed upon by society. What's important is *being healthy*. And to do that you must first accept yourself. The two go hand in hand. To be truly healthy you must first accept your body for what it is. You cannot be otherwise.

Mesomorph

Mesomorphs are to the male community as the hour-glass shape is to females. They gain muscle weight easily and as a result usually have broad shoulders, a thin waist, and boulder-like arms. But they can gain fat too if they aren't careful because their metabolisms aren't as high as their ectomorph brothers. This is the body type that you see portrayed in movies, the one that people on magazine covers claim they have. But do they? This is what magazines tell you you're supposed to look like. But that is simply not the case. You can be sexy and healthy in any of the three body types. Healthy is sexy, but sexy is not always healthy.

Knowledge is power. The reason I'm telling you this is so you know where you come from. There was a fitness book I read that described how to get to the Adonis look regardless of your body type. Basically strangling your body into something it wasn't. Adonis was the name given to the supposedly perfect male body type, what many would consider Michelangelo's David. But if you're trying to twist your body into being what you think it should be instead of accepting it for what it is, you're going about it all wrong. Like I said, all body types have their own strengths and weaknesses. Don't try to give yourself gifts that weren't given you, while stomping out what you have to give to others.

I'm not trying to bash mesomorphs, not at all. However, if you are a mesomorph, it can be easy to neglect your body and think it will just take care of itself. This isn't the case, as all body types have a responsibility to be mindful of what they eat, and to exercise.

Hybrids

There are also combinations of the three body types. They are:

- Ecto-mesomorph
- Endo-mesomorph

Ecto-mesomorph

These body types are usually tall and skinny. Give them the right tools though, and they can gain quite a bit of muscle. It's typically harder for an ecto-mesomorph to gain muscle than their mesomorph brother, however in time it does come. You also have a pretty fast metabolism, which is an added bonus.

Note: Am I only referring to men when I'm talking about the body types? No. Women have these body types too. But they're more obvious to see in men as women have different body proportions.

Endo-mesomorph

People who fit this category are big, but stronger than their endomorph brothers. More muscle means burning more fat, so losing weight is going to be a little easier as well.

There is no perfect body

Let's speculate for a moment that the mesomorph hadn't become the idealized body type. Let's say it was the endomorph. Now, we aren't praising unhealthy habits, rather larger people. We even have our own sport and people praise us for it. We're big and we're strong. Does this sound familiar? They're called sumo wrestlers, and they're treated as celebrities in Japan. Fads come and go, and people's opinions change over time. You too will never be exactly as you are right now and that's okay. Because no matter how you look, as long as you strive to live a healthy life, you're on the right path. Besides, not everyone is attracted to the same thing; some people like short, others tall, etc. Think of an actor or actress who didn't exactly "fit the bill" but you still found attractive in their performance and character.

Chasing after the 'mesomorph' dream is chasing fool's gold. The moment you do you have declared martial law against yourself and have given up your freedom. You've enslaved yourself to the ultimate tyrant, the ego. You say, "I am not worthy so I must make myself worthy." Instead of eating healthy and exercising normally, you starve (or gorge) yourself. All of these things are lies, and create real problems for your health. We are not pieces of granite that need to be sculpted. We are functioning bodies that need to be taken care of and appreciated. You don't go up to an artist and tell them they're wrong because they aren't making the art you like. You don't go up to a dwarf and tell him he's wrong for not being like everyone else. You accept them, or go away. We are all perfect as we are. The trick is to take that acceptance and *then* make ourselves into better people. It's okay to have a role model to look up to, like Rocky, and be inspired by them. It's not okay to beat yourself up and treat yourself badly because you don't look like them. Did you know Sylvester Stallone never competed in professional body-building?[4] There are stories too that he turned down the Bodybuilding Federation numerous times. He knew who he was and how he wanted to look. Instead of turning his body into what was deemed popular at the time, he chose to be who he was. His body is still revered as a work of art.

CHAPTER FOUR

CRITICISM AND KEEPING A CLEAR HEAD

Whether you are having a great day or a bad one, people can pick you up or toss you down, if you let them. You will get upset. You will get angry when someone says something inappropriate to you. But over time and with patience, you can become wiser and more levelheaded when receiving criticism. Obviously, there is a difference between negligible, or destructive, criticism, and positive, or constructive, criticism. We need both to grow, but you can become easier on yourself if you understand the differences between them.

Constructive criticism

All criticism could be considered constructive if you have the right mindset. Whenever you receive criticism, you can stop and ask yourself, "Now, what made this person say that?" If it was rude and poorly thought out then you can come to the conclusion that the person either didn't know what they were talking about, or they were having a bad day. People talk all the time, whether we want them to or not. But you can use a lot of the things they say to your benefit. If someone says you look unhealthy, don't get upset, be honest with yourself. This person may have just saved your life!

> *"A good friend who points out mistakes and imperfections and rebukes evil is to be respected as if he holds the secret to a hidden treasure."* – Buddha

Though this sort of criticism may seem rude or offensive, these can be learning experiences. Take kids for example. Children do not censor themselves; they speak what is on their minds in that moment. Just as it is difficult to avoid children, so too is it difficult to avoid people and their criticisms. The point is not to avoid criticism, rather to let it go. If it is constructive, learn from it, and don't take it personally. Even if it is or might be intended as hurtful, turn it into something positive and see what you can learn from it. Once you recognize that a lot of criticism—even the sort that might appear hurtful and cause great pain in you—can actually be used to your benefit, you can sleep easier and will be more at peace with yourself.

Destructive criticism

I had been working very hard to learn the muscle-up. A muscle-up is an exercise where you pull yourself up to the bar like a pullup, then kip your legs (sort of like a kicking motion) and push yourself up and over the bar. The day finally came, I could feel it. I had been practicing this exercise for so long I was doing it in my sleep. I took my position below the bar. I pulled up, kipped hard, and although it was a bit choppy, I had finally done it, I was up and over the bar! My first official muscle-up. I was super happy and stoked, and was feeling very proud of myself. Just then a couple of Navy Chiefs walked by. They were staring at me and one of them scoffed, "Pff, I could do that too if I was that small and skinny."

I was crushed. It was like someone had handed me a bowling ball on cloud nine and I was plummeting towards earth. They had no idea how much hard work I put in. All of the mornings I had woken up early to head to the gym and practice. All of the disappointment and embarrassment from not being able to perform the exercise; pulling myself up to the bar and being unable to push myself over the top. But I choose not to get upset because I know that they had no idea what they were talking about. They didn't know how much time and energy I had put into mastering that exercise. Harmful criticism is ignorant criticism.

When we get angry or upset, jealous or embarrassed, we talk before we think. We say the first thing that comes to mind to defend our egos. It seems much easier to sputter out some kind of defense than to suck it up and keep quiet. But responding defensively only fuels the other person. It is best to turn the other cheek and go back to working on yourself. I'd rather spend my energy doing push-ups than arguing with an ignoramus.

Become neutral

When it comes to taking criticism from others, it's best to remain neutral. What does this mean? Does it mean to scoff at people who laugh at you? Does it mean to ignore others? No, it simply means to not take anyone's words as a measure of how well you're doing. Simply put, don't take what people say to you personally, whether it is negative or positive. This might sound narcissistic, but don't take words of praise to heart. Because if you rely on what other people say as your primary source of motivation, then you're only going to make yourself susceptible when they say things that are less than positive.

Nothing to do with you

I had a teacher in high school who told us a story about his sick mother. She had been diagnosed with Alzheimer's. One day, as her condition worsened, he stood by her bed, hoping she might recognize him and say something meaningful. As he stood there, she finally opened her eyes.

He waited anxiously for what she was about to say.

She turned her head to him and her eyes became wide. "You're a vampire!"

At that moment he ran out of the room and burst into tears, but then he pulled himself together, "This is the disease, not my mother."

And with that he was able to calm himself down and return to the room.

I would say many of us in our daily lives take things personally that we really shouldn't. Let's take a look at my teacher's situation. Because he was able to step away from the problem, he was able to understand its true meaning.

As emotional human beings, we want to look at a situation like this and say, "Oh my dear mother, she doesn't remember me at all! She just called me a vampire! Oh, woe is me! Woe is me!"

Instead of looking at problems and taking them personally, let's look at them constructively. This way we can reevaluate and see what is really going on.

You'll find that sometimes it doesn't even have anything to do with you. The person may just be upset. Maybe they broke up with their girlfriend. There are so many factors, but none that you should take to heart.

If you know you have been exercising, even if someone comes up to you and calls you a fat slob, you can hold your head high. You don't have to throw a chair at them. You don't even have to blink because you know the truth.

One of my favorite quotes comes from Buddha:

"Believe nothing, no matter where you read it, no matter who said it, even if I have said it, unless it agrees with your own reason and your own common sense."

CHAPTER FIVE

WHAT IS FITNESS?

What exactly makes a person fit? Is it the size of their waist? Their biceps? Is it the percentage of body fat they have? Most people misconstrue what fitness is, and it's not difficult to blame them. Every day we are bombarded with articles and headlines from the "best" magazines telling us what fitness is. But let's be honest, most of what we *think* we know about fitness, especially in today's American culture, is not simply misguided, it's wrong.

We live in a world where people believe being healthy means looking sexy, that the two are somehow one and the same. And while looking good is often the result of taking care of your body, it is not always what comes first, or as Dr. Phil would say, "It's the old case of the tail wagging the dog." We choose "sexy" first and healthy second. As I often repeat, people will do whatever it takes to have a "sexy" body. But a "sexy" body is not always a healthy body.

Fitness is not just about having six-pack abs or boulder-sized biceps. It's not simply about having three percent body fat or being able to bench press five hundred pounds. Being truly fit means being able to take whatever life throws at you and persevere. It means that when all the gimmicks and fads are taken away and it's just you standing cold and naked at the bottom of a cave with nothing but the rats to keep you company, you have deep down inside you, the fire to persevere.

So what is fitness? What the heck is it?

For us beginners (and maybe those of us who aren't) let's break it down. These are the three basic (and yet very important) pillars of fitness.

Cardio endurance

Cardio, or cardiovascular endurance is the ability of your heart and lungs to fuel your body with oxygen.[5] Sounds very important. In fact, sounds like one of the *most* important things. So then how come every time I'm in the gym, the treadmills are almost entirely vacant? I believe that health begins with your heart. That's why it's the center of your body. It's the nucleus of this whole mechanism. If you're not taking care of your heart, i.e., you're not pumping it with life-sustaining oxygen, then you're wasting your time. If you don't take care of the heart, if you don't take care of your cardio, then everything else falls apart. Do you know I avoided running like the plague because I was more concerned about how I looked, more worried about the calories I might burn (remember I'm an ectomorph) than I was about taking care of my heart? That's ridiculous! But that's what a lot of us do every day.

Flexibility

I hated stretching. Hated it. Thought it was pointless. All I wanted to do was exercise. But like a good boy I would give five minutes to a light stretch. Your body is not invincible. It's very durable, but it's not invincible. The things that you're asking your body to do are above its normal workload: lifting heavy things, moving weights around, etc. Stretching is done to prevent injuries, but we snuff at it. It's important to think of your body as cold taffy. What happens if you take a hammer to cold taffy? It shatters. But when you warm up that taffy and hit it with the same hammer, what happens? It absorbs the impact. Every day you work out and perform a hard job, you are smashing your body with a large hammer. But we don't want to be bothered with stretching. That's sissy stuff only girls in yoga do.

True strength though is flexibility because flexibility is durability. If you're constantly going to work on your body without laying down the law, you're just asking for trouble. I'll share with you a story about something stupid I did. And you can bet it involves the lack of stretching!

One day long ago, in a land far, far away, I was in a gym on a crowded base. Today—that day—happened to be leg day. Hooray! Everybody's favorite day. Well on that particular day, I was in a hurry. I didn't feel I needed to stretch my legs, especially for a muscle group as tiny and forgetful as my calves. So there I am sitting on the calf-raise machine. I put extra weights on the side cuz I ain't no chump. Just loaded them up there. Then went to town. Up down, up down, up down, up pop. Woah, what was that? The scary thing was, it wasn't a balloon pop, oh no, it was like a quiet leak of air, a deflation. I didn't think anything of it. Have you ever done something so bad, that you quickly pretended—tried to convince yourself—that it didn't exist, or it actually hadn't happened? Like trying to sneak backwards through time, "Well that was close!" I walked off the platform and went home for the day. But deep down inside I knew something was wrong. A few days later, I had an erroneous limp. It was like walking on a flat tire. I had blown a tendon underneath my foot. I can't say for sure because I'm not a doctor (and I never went to medical) but it may have been the plantar fascia. Wouldn't you know it, I had a deployment coming up. And I limped the entire cruise. I tell you this story as a warning: not stretching has severe consequences. But why is stretching important, besides preventing injury? As I said, true strength lies in flexibility. Picture rubber bands. Alone, they snap easily, but together they're stronger. Creating flexibility creates a union in your body, a familiarity between different muscle groups and parts. And unity is stronger than alone.

Strength

Oh yes, strength. But where does strength come from? And what is strength? I'm going to share with you something that you may not know, certainly I had not known it when I first started working out: All muscular people are not strong. Let me say that again: ALL MUSCULAR PEOPLE ARE NOT STRONG. But Dave, they are all strong, aren't they? I mean, look at those muscles! Some of them are strong, but not all of them. Just like we said about how not everyone sexy is healthy, well not everyone muscular is strong. There are a few reasons for this. The first is they may just be taking supplements, getting double the results for half the work. The second is, they're not working out for strength, they're just working out to look better. Now, there's nothing inherently wrong with this, but there it is. And finally: they may be strong, but their strength is only skin deep. Let me explain.

Where does true strength come from? Seriously? Where does it come from? *Well, it comes from lifting heavy things, of course!* Does it? What is lifting those heavy things? *The muscles!* Yes. *And, the skeleton?* Yes. *And, erm.* Deeper. I'll give you a hint, we mentioned one of them earlier. Tendons and ligaments! Tendons and ligaments are the foundation of strength. They are what true strength is built on. But most people have this backwards, they believe that strength starts with the muscles in. Actually it's the opposite. The muscles are the last leg of strength. The first leg is ligaments and tendons, then the bones, and finally the muscles. That's why people who lift heavy will usually hit a plateau. Why? Because they're not going deep with their tendons and ligaments. Then how do you build strength from the ground up? There are a few ways, but one of the most effective is calisthenics, or the use of bodyweight exercises. This is because the body is working with the perfect amount of resistance against the perfect amount of weight, and that's the keyword: resistance. When I was younger, my dad had a Bow flex in his basement. Remember those? I used to work out on it all the time, but I thought it was a completely useless machine, I mean, where're the weights?! Little did I know, that was one of the best ways to start out exercising, especially for a young person.

Resistance creates strength because resistance builds from the ground up: first the tendons and ligaments, then the skeletal system, then the muscles. You know the saying, you're only as strong as your weakest link? It's not because the weakest link is weak, it's because the weakest link is usually neglected or ignored. The weakest link is actually the strongest (or at least has the potential to be). Nothing is more neglected, and yet more important, than the tendons and ligaments in terms of strength. Because that is where true strength lies.

CHAPTER SIX

EATING RIGHT

In his book *Sly Moves*, Sylvester Stallone talks about the many different diets and why they don't work. Diets come from a lack of understanding about the body. Many are created by doctors and I believe that's where the problem lies. When you overthink things, commonsense fades and you miss the big picture. I think we complicate things just so we can feel smart. But real intelligence doesn't come from complicating simple things, it comes from simplifying complicated things. We've confused the hell out of each other, and that's why diets don't work.

Eating right

Do we remember what it means to eat right? Have you heard of this before? Not dieting, eating well-balanced food and giving your body the vitamins and nutrients it needs. What I'm talking about is how we can make eating simpler. Not everyone has money to buy, or access to, the healthiest foods. You don't have to shop at the fanciest stores and buy the most expensive fruits and vegetables. You don't have to buy organic this and organic that. You don't have to buy brown eggs dipped in olive oil. All you need is common sense. If you normally eat sugary cereal, why not replace it with oatmeal? If you normally buy pudding, why not instead buy yogurt? Take a look at what you have in your pantry. How much has been sitting there forever? Throw away what doesn't work and get back to basics.

Eating right happens in small steps. It happens when you decide to no longer buy fatty chips. It happens when you decide to use a healthy alternative to butter, perhaps margarine. Eating right doesn't have to be complicated, you just have to cut out the noise. Mother Nature gave us everything we need to live, and all of it is in your local grocery store. It may not be the best of the best, but it's only as good as you make it. Eat well-balanced food, give your body the nutrients it needs, and stop doing diets. Everything you need is right in front of you.

So many choices!

A big reason why eating right is intimidating is

because we think that in order to eat well, we must be master chefs. If you are not a cook, all those prep sheets and recipes can be daunting. But eating well doesn't require you to be a cook; you don't need to create fancy meals.

Another misconception is you have to eat a different meal every day. But that's just luxury. If you want to eat the same meal, all the time, then go ahead. More than likely though, you'll get bored. That's why there are different options. I personally eat the same things most of the time. A lot of people do. So why not eat the same healthy meals, instead of the same unhealthy ones? If you are a cook, why not use your powers for good? There are more healthy delicious meals you can make than you can imagine. And most of that just comes from supplementing different ingredients.

Listening to your stomach

Am I hungry?

Do I need to eat right now?

When will I be eating again?

These are all questions you need to be asking yourself. Too many times we think we're starving to death when we're just bored. When was the last time you ate? When will you be eating again? Does your work have you eating at specific times of the day, or are you able to eat whenever you want? Organize your meals. If you know you won't be eating for some time, plan ahead and prep. If you're not hungry in the morning, wait until you are. Learn your eating habits. Don't force-feed yourself. Remember, common sense.

Pseudo hunger

The problem is when you eat just to eat. I know we get bored, upset, and lonely, but junk food only makes things worse. They say when you're hungry at night, you're just thirsty. So drink a glass of water. If you're still hungry, eat something light. If you recognize you're just bored, do something that takes your mind off of food—call a friend, read a book, etc.

Mindful eating

Perhaps you've heard of mindful walking. What about mindful eating? When we eat, we really like to make an event of it. We've got to have our favorite TV show on, our feet propped up, and wearing our favorite pajamas. This probably comes from when we were kids and our parents let us eat cereal while we watched our morning cartoons. But after you're done eating, did you even eat? Did you taste the food and recognize when you were no longer hungry? When you juggle eating with a distraction, such as watching television, you take out the very act of eating. The food just disappears.

When you eat, try to stay away from TV, put down your phone, and just eat. And if you can, eat with others. It makes the experience much more enjoyable.

Before and after you exercise

If you don't already have something in your stomach, eat before you work out. You'll hear people say, *You must eat this much, this long before you exercise.* But it just comes down to listening. If I ate not long ago, I ask myself, *am I hungry? Do I have the energy to get this done?* If the answer is no, then I eat something. If it's in the morning, I'll have a light meal and maybe some coffee. Nothing fancy, just enough to get me going. But not too much that it slows me down. Then, when I'm done exercising, I'm hungry again. It's a win/win.

My older brother and I used to joke after working out:

Hurry, you've got t-minus thirty minutes to eat before your muscles deteriorate!

The reality is, sometimes you're just not hungry when you're done exercising. Especially if you're still full from the meal you had earlier. It is never a good idea to force-feed yourself; there's a reason why you're not hungry. It's the body's way of saying, *"Relax, just let me recoup a little before you start cramming food down our throat."* Sometimes I'm starving after I exercise, other times I have to wait until I'm hungry. This can be upwards to an hour; not usually past that though. While I don't believe you have to eat immediately after you exercise, I do believe you should feed your muscles as soon as you're hungry.

Food psychology

If I tell myself I cannot eat something, my desire to eat that thing increases tenfold. But if I give myself the freedom to choose what I want, I am ten times more likely to make a better decision. When I was doing my amateur bodybuilding routine, I was bulking and cutting. Bulking is when you eat more calories than you're used to in order to gain mass. Cutting is when you eat fewer calories than you're used to in order to cut fat. This had come to be known as Yoyo dieting in the few years after it was introduced. Normally I would say it was called this because the people who were doing it were yoyo's, but it's probably just because of the up and down motion of a yoyo. When I was bulking, do you think I loved shoving food down my throat? I hated it. Why? It's simple psychology. Because I had to. I was forcing myself. And when I was cutting, I was starving.

I have since cut out Yoyo dieting. Not simply because it is bad for my metabolism, but because I don't believe in it anymore. When I allow myself to make a decision, I'm the one in charge, not food. And when I'm the one in charge, I usually make the better decision.

CHAPTER SEVEN

WATER, WATER, WATER

Why do we hear how amazing water is and never drink it? Water is the most important thing your body needs, not just to function properly, but to function at all.

We are water, water is energy

When I was on deployment, the most important thing I did for myself was drink lots of water. I was drinking probably fifteen bottles a day, but I needed it. I was working long hours in a hot, cramped environment. I discovered it does more than just hydrate you, it energizes and keeps you focused. The body is made up of roughly sixty percent water, and the heart and brain are over seventy.[6] It is our vehicle's gasoline. But it's amazing how much we turn to coffee and energy drinks when water is plenty on its own. It's the magic elixir! It will give you energy you didn't know you had, keep your mind sharp, and keep your organs running smoothly.

Waking up and before eating

I usually drink a cup of water when I wake up. The body has been without it for a long time and is dehydrated. I drink it to replenish my internal structure. I also drink a cup, or half a cup, before a meal. It clears the pipes and is good for digestion.

Water and exercise

There's a fine line between being dehydrated and drinking too much water when exercising. Some workouts are harder than others, and sometimes we exercise outside. You don't want to get sick by drinking too much water, but you don't want to pass out either from not drinking enough. The rule of thumb is to sip, not gulp.

But if you ever feel lightheaded or nauseous while exercising, sit down, breathe, and take a few sips. If you're still not feeling well, call it a day. This has happened to me a few times. Your safety is more important than the workout. I don't want you passing out and grilling like a pancake in the sun.

Extra-lytes

A lot of people drink sports drinks because of the

taste. When you drink them while not active, you consume more electrolytes than your body needs. Sports drinks are meant to replenish you in ways that water can't, but the situations you need them are few. Unless you're overheated or sweating profusely, drinking them on their own does more harm than good. It just sloshes around in your gut.

Soda

I don't need to explain to you why soda is bad. So instead I'd like to share with you a story my sixth-grade science teacher told our class:

"Imagine taking a shower in a sugary, brown substance. Imagine getting out of that shower, drying off, with the towel sticking to you. You spend the rest of the day smelling and cooking in the sun, probably a few flies buzzing around you. Imagine what that feels like. That's what you do to the inside of your body when you drink soda."

CHAPTER EIGHT

CAFFEINE AND NAPS

Like many great things, too much caffeine can be bad for you, and this can certainly be the case for caffeine and exercise as well. The body sometimes needs a kick start like a car, other times it has more than enough energy. But how can you tell?

Your body brings its own energy

Imagine a cup filling with water. The cup is your body, the water is energy. You can only pour so much water into the cup before it starts to overflow. In situations like exercise, your body brings its own energy, similar to the kind our ancestors acquired when getting ready to run from a predator: your heart starts pumping blood faster, your palms start to sweat. But if we drink too much caffeine, we can cause that cup to overflow. When that happens, you get things like the shakes and a much higher than desired heart rate. I call it stripping the car. You know those toy cars you wind up and let go? When you wind them back too far they snap, what we used to call stripping. That's what you do to your body when you drink too much caffeine, you wind it up past its breaking point.

Is your mood just low?

Say you come home from work and are agitated about something that happened that day. You say to yourself, "I don't feel like exercising." But you're stubborn and drink some caffeine anyway. It wasn't your energy that was low, it was your mood. You were at a cool fifty percent and just added twenty. Now when you start exercising and your body brings its own energy to the table, your heart rate goes through the roof.

Caffeine as training wheels

Caffeine is good for a push. It's like training wheels before you let little Timmy go. But it's important to feel your energy levels and be wise when drinking any caffeine before you exercise.

The summit of Caffeine Mountain

At some point you're going to drink too much caffeine and reach the summit of Caffeine Mountain; pitch a tent and take a nap. No more caffeine is going to help. Because nothing is worse than being too tired to do anything, and yet too wired to sleep. A nap is what you need, not more caffeine.

The magic of naps

There is only so much caffeine you can drink, you'll reach a point where it no longer serves you. Find a comfortable place to sit and rest with your back against it for ten to fifteen minutes. I usually cross my arms and tilt my head. Sometimes you'll sleep longer, others shorter. I don't set a timer, I just let my mind wake naturally. Just don't lay down like you're going to bed. When you do that, instead of sleeping for a few minutes, you'll fall asleep for hours because your body thinks it's time for bed. It shuts the whole system down. When you sleep upright, only the brain rests, like a computer going into sleep mode. You'll wake up refreshed and ready to go.

Let go

The first few seconds of a nap are the best, but then your mind starts to chatter: *The fight you had with your boyfriend, plans you had for dinner, taking the car to the shop.* There's so much going on that by the time the nap is over, you haven't rested at all. Close your eyes and let go. Just let that rhythmically run through your mind, "*Let go. Let go.*" Feel it throughout your entire body. Focus on rest. Eventually this will put you into a deep state where you will feel your heart and mind start to relax.

Like a cat

In Konstantin Stanislavski's book, *An Actor Prepares*, he talks about letting go of tightness in the body. He used to walk like a plank while on stage and to solve this, he watched his cat. It was completely loose when sleeping—not a single muscle in its body was tight. He picked the cat up and looked at the imprint it made on the bed. It sank like an anchor. When you're tight, the stiffest parts of your body sink deeper. Do a mental sweep of your body and look for places that are tight. For the cat, it was all even, meaning it had no tightness in its body. It was resting completely. And as you may know, picking up a sleeping cat is like picking up a melting piece of taffy.

CHAPTER NINE

EXERCISE SUPPLEMENTS

When I did my amateur bodybuilding routine, I was rolling in exercise supplements morning, noon, and night. It was all I thought about:

What do I have to take today?

How much?

How many times?

No wonder some bodybuilders go off the deep end. There's this story of a young bodybuilder who was in his priming phase, which means he was putting on the finishing touches before a contest. His physique was great but he was on edge. As he was walking to the gym from the parking lot some joker said, "Hey bro, do you even lift?" The bodybuilder stormed back to his truck, grabbed a gun, and shot the other man in the leg. Thankfully the story is said to be fake, but it still shows the dark side of how obsessed we can become with exercise.[7] And supplements can become a big part of that obses-sion. It certainly was with me.

Note: In this chapter when I talk about supple-ments, I am talking about *exercise supplements*, not nutritional or dietary supplements prescribed by a doctor or sold behind the counter at pharmacies.

Should you take them?

Walk into any supplement store and your head will spin. There are fat-burning supplements, weight gain supplements, creatine, etc. There is a lot of pressure to take exercise supplements. Remember when I said exercise is a journey? Supplements promise that great American appeal: NOW. You don't gain fifty pounds of muscle, or lose fifty pounds of weight overnight. Do it naturally, that's where long-term health lives. Watch what you eat, go for walks, cut out smoking, etc. Unless you are a high-performing professional athlete, there is no supplement you need to take.

Hulk smash

On my second deployment, I made friends with a guy I'll call John. He saw that I liked to work out and gave me a container of pre-workout powder. I thought, what the heck, I'll give it a shot. That evening after work, I took a spoonful right before exercise. It was like lightning running through my body. You get this charge of energy that feels like a thousand needles under your skin. I realized I had a problem when, after two hours of heavy lifting, I still wasn't tired. I laid in my rack for the wonderful four hours I was provided. I don't think I even blinked. After what seemed like an eternity, I got up to go to work. Later I crashed. Thank God for the head (bathroom). Sailors are renowned for being able to sleep in the most unique of places.

The cost

Investing in exercise supplements will burn a hole in your pocket. Spending on peanut butter sandwiches would be a better use of your money. When I first started exercising, I truly believed I needed a protein shake after my workout. It's funny now looking back, but I seriously thought that this was the only way my muscles would grow. And people still ask me what kind of protein they should be taking. I try to put myself back in the mindset of someone just starting. It's a shame that this is the story we're told on how to fuel our bodies after we exercise. The answer is none, unless it's made with real ingredients like milk, nuts, and fruit. Get real food into your body. There's also the cost to your health. Protein shakes on the market are mostly artificial gunk made up in a lab somewhere, pumped with sugar and empty calories. Personally, I like to know what kind of things I'm putting into my body. If I can't even pronounce the ingredients written on the label, I probably shouldn't be consuming it at all.

I stopped taking exercise supplements years ago, and it was one of the best decisions I made concerning exercise. I was spending hundreds of dollars a month and hours a week worrying about them and it took a hold of my life. Getting rid of exercise supplements saved me time, money, and headache. And there are more important things in my life to worry about. The reason supplements are so popular is because they promise quick results. And they try to make you believe that they are the only way to get those results. But long-term health doesn't come in a bottle. And when you take something because you believe it will instantly solve all of your problems, you've missed the point. Health is a journey, but supplements promise a destination.

Hulk smash— again

After reading some article online about how male testosterone has significantly diminished over thousands of years, I decided it was best to get my testosterone levels up too (I make sporadic decisions like this sometimes). I went to the supplement store on base and bought myself a bottle of testosterone booster. I'm surprised they sold that stuff there.

A warning against testosterone boosters: These supplements cause irritability, aggression, and anxiousness. I was taking these suckers before work and saying things like, "If so and so ever talks to me like that again, I'll toss 'em overboard!" I didn't notice my aggression until a friend pointed it out to me, "Man, what happened to you? You're salty as heck!" I laughed, but it was the first time I could see what he was talking about. I thought something was off. This wasn't me talking, it was all the extra testosterone. I decided to cut out the supplement and haven't used it since.

The reason I told you this story is because most supplements don't tell you the side effects. Even things like creatine are banned from military training because it stores water in the muscles, leaving you dehydrated.[8] It also causes cramping and diarrhea—side effects in the field you don't want happening.

Good old fashion

When people start exercising, they generally do it

for one of two reasons: to build muscle or to lose weight. But before they even hit the gym, they wonder how they'll do this. They think, there must be some magic formula hidden from the masses. *If I can only find this elixir, I can be like the people on the magazines.* Most people believe that just because they're taking supplements— even if they're training poorly— they're training well. The truth is, supplements fuel all of the wrong reasons why you should be working out. If you want to gain muscle or lose weight, the secret formula is food. Quit shopping in the supplement store and start shopping in the grocery store. Want to really feed your muscles? Eat some grilled chicken and go for seconds. There is no replacement for actual food—it says so on the supplement container!

Chapter Ten

When Should You Exercise?

We're all busy people with hectic work schedules that fluctuate every day. When are you supposed to exercise? Here are three different scenarios that I have personally adopted, each with their own unique benefits.

In the morning or before work

In the morning your energy levels are at their highest. After a night of sleep, your body is fully recharged. Even if you need a small cup of coffee to wake up, you will still have the best energy levels. Morning is also a great time to exercise because once you're done, you don't have to think about it anymore for the rest of the day. It also energizes you and puts a smile on your face. Nothing makes me feel better than knowing that when I go home I can just relax and do what I want.

In the afternoon or during break

If you find yourself squeezed for time, you could always take a quick lunch and punch in a quick workout. It doesn't have to be some complex or elaborate affair. In fact, some of my best workouts have been quick. When your brain understands you have only a short amount of time to get something done, it will work harder to compensate and you will be more focused. Do you think you would work out harder if you were given three hours to exercise or only one?

In the evening or after work

Exercising in the evening can be great because it's an amazing stress reliever, especially if you've had a bad day. Is your boss giving you problems? These pushups are for him! A big complaint I used to hear from sailors on deployment was, "If I work out before bed, I can't go to sleep." The idea is that after working out you're energized. I don't attribute this to the workout so much as to other things:

1. You're still feeling any caffeine you drank.
2. Your workout just wasn't hard enough.

I would recommend staying away from drinking caffeine before you exercise if you have this problem. Or just working out in the morning or afternoon instead.

Pros/cons

All of these times to exercise are great in their own way; each has its benefits and none are better than the others. I use all three of them myself, changing it up when I get bored or tired of the same routine. Everyone does from time to time. You may exercise in the morning for six months and be fine with it, and then one day wake up and are not feeling it. So do we give up? Of course not! We change our routine. If you had to eat the same thing every day, even if you loved it, eventually you'd lose your taste for it. It's about having options and knowing that you're not cemented to one time of day.

Chapter Eleven

Our Exercise Tool Kit

There are a few things you need to bring with you when you work out. Some of them I consider necessary, and others are dependent on your needs. Let's take a look at them and see what we want in our arsenal (and a few things we don't).

Exercise partners

If you have someone who can motivate you and push you, they might be a good exercise partner. Having a friend to keep you accountable can be great, but you need to make sure that you aren't relying on them too much because if you take them away and you're lost, you'll have a harder time exercising. Let's take a look at some of the pros and cons of having an exercise partner.

Pros:

- Helps motivate you

- Pushes you
- Keeps you accountable

Cons:

- You can become dependent
- Does not know what is best for YOUR exercise routine
- Can be temperamental/unpredictable

In the end, it might not be in your best interest to have someone you fully rely on to exercise. I personally have never chosen to have a workout partner. I do not mind helping people during my workout, but I'm mostly like a pair of training wheels. I'll give them a push, point them in the right direction, and let go. I am not saying you should never have a workout partner. If you need one to help you grow, or if you know someone who is also starting out, then it might be helpful for both of you to exercise together. But never become dependent on someone to exercise. I've heard too many stories of people giving up because their partner gave up.

Music

Listening to music can be a great way to spend a workout. It pumps you up, keeps you motivated, and entertains you. There is nothing like enjoying yourself while getting fit. Music can be wonderful, but if you're not careful, it can become a distraction. If you find yourself pausing an entire workout every time a song ends to search for a new song, you've got a problem because now the workout is no longer the central focus, your music is.

A guy I worked with absolutely REFUSED to work out if he didn't have his music with him. And do you know what happened? His iPod broke. In the middle of deployment. And he was stubborn as a bull. *"Nope, can't do it. Won't do it."* If you put too much pressure on something that, if you were to lose it, ruins your entire motivation to do something, it's a problem. Don't do that to music. Let it be a motivator, but don't become dependent on it as your sole reason for working out.

Quiet time

I work out mostly without music. As much as I enjoy listening to it, it becomes a distraction. I've exercised for so long that I've reached a point where I'm subconsciously monitoring, tracking, and evaluating my workouts. It's like a tiny whisper that says to me, *"Do it this way, not that way. Add another set here. Do you want to do more reps on this next exercise? Okay, we'll do that."* When I'm listening to music during a workout, I'm half paying attention. But when it's just me and the workout, and no music, I focus entirely on what I'm doing. This helps me to get more work done, instead of just throwing weights around or going through the motions. It's hard but it's worth it. And over time you can develop such a relationship with your workouts, that you'll wonder how you were ever able to get through an entire workout before. People listen to music when they work out because they want to be motivated. But if you can get to a place where your workout comes from inside you, not outside, then you'll become a very powerful force.

Music can be great, if you don't abuse it. If you simply cannot exercise without it, I ask you to reevaluate what you are doing. Because the moment something happens and your music is gone, the rug gets pulled out from under you. Let music be an enjoyable addition, not a crutch. Find the balance between listening to it and not listening to it. A buddy of mine used to sing under his breath while on deployment. I asked him about it once, wondering why he didn't just get an iPod like everyone else. He said, *"Brother, the best iPod I have is in my head."*

Exercise notebook

This is it. The Big Kahuna. The Big Lebowski. This is THE SINGLE MOST IMPORTANT PIECE OF EQUIPMENT YOU NEED IN YOUR EXERCISE BAG. Walking into your workout without something to log your progress is like taking a college course and not getting any credits for it. You can rely on memory, but a notebook gives you much more than that. A notebook is the blueprint of your fitness.

All of your strengths and weaknesses are in that notebook, all of the things you're working towards, all of the little critiques and notes you write to yourself. I believe a notebook is the difference between a lifelong learner and someone who quits.

It doesn't have to be anything fancy, just a cheap, small, two hundred page or so notebook you can find at any dollar store. A notebook is about more than just logging progress, it's about logging YOUR progress. And just like your identity, your progress will be different than everyone else's. You couldn't cheat off of your friend's notebook even if you lost yours. Yours is only identifiable to you. It's your thumbprint.

Some things your notebook could contain:

- Exercises
- Progressions
- Personal side notes (Perhaps how you will accomplish a harder exercise)
- Inspirational quotes
- Words of wisdom from you
- Epiphanies
- Anything else you feel will help improve the quality of your workouts

Miscellaneous

Here are some other things you may want to consider when going to the gym. They're basic, but no less important:

- Water bottle (so you aren't always running to the fountain)
- Grip gloves (if you have sweaty palms or there's no grip powder)
- Hoodie/sweats (good for warm-ups and when it's cold)
- Light towel (for sweating)

- Heavy towel (if you're taking a shower at the gym)
- Toiletries (for your shower)
- Shower shoes (you don't want your bare feet touching that floor)
- Gym Bag (so you can carry all that crap)

Chapter Twelve

Lost Training Secrets

Walk into any gym and look around, then leave and come back in five years. Chances are you will see the same people doing the same thing. Avid gym go-ers have been saying that for years, but it holds some truth. It was certainly my experience. You don't want to be doing the same thing years from now, you want to be improving yourself and your workouts. This isn't just about getting bigger or leaner; improving your workout can mean any number of things, from increases in flexibility, to better form, or a stronger cardiovascular system.

Mind/muscle link

Most of us think of exercise as solely training our bodies, but there's something more important happening if we only become quiet and listen. In Brooks Kubik's book, *Dinosaur Bodyweight Training*, Kubik refers to something he calls the *mind/muscle link*. It simply means connecting the mind to your body through exercise. Let's take a novice and ask him to do a set of pushups. He goes to the ground and just flops up and down like a fish out of water. Boom, boom, boom.

But when you do a push-up, what is being worked? The chest, the shoulders, the triceps, even the biceps and entire midsection. Your calves too if you're digging them into the ground. Almost everything, but you have to be focused on what you're doing. A good way to make that connection is by getting into position of the exercise you are doing, and then holding that position for one minute. It's almost like doing yoga. Hold the position, don't move, and don't do any repetitions. Just feel the muscles, and try to locate each one, even the tiny ones. Do this every day as a warmup before your workout until you create a connection. When you do a push-up, feel the push-up, don't just flop up and down like a fish. Be methodical. Imagine you're filling up one of those honey bears with honey, that's what you're doing. You're filling the mold.

Milking

Milking refers to using an exercise until it no longer serves you. That could mean lifting twenty-pound dumbbells of bicep curls for three weeks; they're not too light and they're not too heavy, and you're seeing and feeling results. But we're always comparing ourselves to others; everything's a competition, so why waste time in the gym lifting light weights? Look at the guy over there curling sixties! We sacrifice what works to save face. Milking is the meaning of the phrase, *if it ain't broke, don't fix it.* If something is working, keep doing it. When that something doesn't anymore, stop. How do you know when it's no longer working for you? It will start to feel boring and monotonous, and you'll no longer see or feel results; you'll feel like you're just spinning your wheels.

When I got off my bodybuilding routine, I had a golden era in my exercise. I would do countless pushups, pull-ups, sit-ups, etc., until I couldn't anymore. My body was indulging in a smorgasbord after years of lifting weights. As much as I didn't want it to end though, the phase came to pass. It was a great milking period, but all good things must come to an end. And when that happens, it's time to move on to something harder.

Progression

Progression is what happens when you perform harder exercises. It's when you've reached a point in exercise where you're too comfortable. Once an exercise becomes too easy, it's time to move on to something more difficult. A few more pushups here, a new level of difficulty there, etc. If you do five pushups in your first week, you might find that you can do eight pushups in the second week, and twelve pushups in the third. But progression doesn't mean you forget easier exercises for the rest of your life. You can use them as warm-ups or on days when you're not feeling one hundred percent. Now, it's important to know that when I say an exercise becomes too easy, I don't mean that you've been doing it for a few days. Progression happens over weeks, months, even years. It's a good thing. There is always a way to progress, and you will find a way that best suits you, whether that means a progression in the number of reps, or a progression to a more difficult exercise. It's up to you.

The alphabet

Remember we said fitness is a journey? Think of that journey as being on the alphabet. When you're going through the alphabet, you don't jump from A *alllllllll* the way to Z. You go letter by letter, from *A* to *B* to *C*, etc. And because fitness is a journey and not a destination, you:

1. Are always somewhere on the alphabet.
2. Understand "Z" does not exist.

3. Don't get upset if you aren't on say, letter F.
4. Commend yourself for being on the alphabet at all. Some people look at it and say, no thank you!

Invisible membrane

I used to think that to be a great runner, I just had to keep running. But no matter how much I ran, I wasn't getting any better. It's not enough to be like the Energizer Bunny and just keep going, you have to push through the resistance if you want to get better. First I start in a light jog, then I pick up the pace. I have to push. My body wants to cruise, but if I want to run harder, I have to fight through the resistance. I imagine running inside an invisible membrane. At cruising speed, I'm sitting in it, nice and cozy. I may push against it every once in a while, but nothing too serious that I break through it. If I want to break through that darn thing, I have to push. I push a little harder than yesterday. But I don't wipe myself out. It is uncomfortable. But the next time, it is less uncomfortable. And the next time, and the next time. I'm not simply talking about running here, I understand that running is not for everyone. The invisible membrane is about anything in your workout, anywhere you can give yourself a little more to. I'm not saying to strain or hurt yourself, but are you giving it enough, or are you walking away early leaving a little something on the table?

Chapter Thirteen

Different Types of Training

There are many different types of training out there, but the purpose of this book is not to persuade you in any one direction. You need to find what works for you and what you enjoy best. Just be mindful of others' way of training. If you get bored, mix it up. But find something that speaks to you and stick with it. If you dig many small holes, you'll never dig one deep. This is a general overview of some of the different exercise methods out there.

Come down off your pedestal

When you're really good at something, it's easy to think that you're the best. But when you do, you rob yourself of humility, which makes you miss bigger things. The ego closes the mind. There's always going to be someone who's better than you at something. That's why it's important to see the other ways in which people train.

Weightlifting

This is probably the most widely used form of exercise in the world. When done properly, weightlifting can be a great way to build strength. Unfortunately, a lot of people don't know what they're doing with the weights. To properly train with weights, you must be mindful, as with everything. Don't just lift the weights up and down, be methodical. If you can't lift a weight without contorting your body into strange shapes, you must go with a lighter weight. My opinion would be to go with a weight that you are able to perform eight reps in strict form with. That means keeping a straight body and not shaking all over. If you want to lift heavier, go for a weight that you can lift well for five reps. But be mindful and be careful. My strong opinion is that no one should even touch weights without two years of strict calisthenics training. But that's just me.

Kettlebell

Kettlebell training is versatile, builds strength, and gets your heart pumping. But what the heck is it? The beautiful thing about kettlebell training, as opposed to regular weightlifting, is that it's all about controlling the weight. When you're lifting weights, you go for reps and sets, lifting up and down to get blood in the muscles. With kettlebell, you're focused more on skeletal strength. To give you an idea of what I'm talking about, grab a heavy book and hold it out in front of you for thirty seconds, then slowly lower it to the ground. In kettlebell training, it's about stability and control. When you have the weight in your hands, you don't throw it around like a rag doll, you control it. If the weight is in front of you, you control the downward motion. This creates amazing strength and is the reason it's so popular.

Calisthenics

When I hit a wall with my weight training routine, a colleague of mine introduced me to a few books I mentioned in the introduction. I had been training with weights for some years, but this promised exercise without gyms and weights. I was fascinated because the hours I was working were many, and the hole in the wall they called a gym was too crowded after work to do anything. Calisthenics is using your body as your exercise tool. There are no weights, no fancy pieces of equipment you need to buy. It's just you, the ground, a wall, and hopefully a pullup bar somewhere. Unfortunately, this type of training faded into the background when weights became popular, but all of the best strongmen in the early nineteenth century had some form of hard calisthenics training. What makes it unique is that it's a natural form of training and it's simple. You don't see lions or bears lifting weights in the wild, they use what nature gave them. When doing pushups or squats, you're using the perfect amount of weight to perform the perfect amount of reps. Unlike weights, you increase the level of difficulty through different positioning, or harder variations. For example, if regular pushups become too easy, you may start performing what is called a diamond pushup, where the hands are close together to form the shape of a diamond. The possibilities are end-less, all you need is a little imagination. Calisthenics trains your whole body: nervous system, skeletal system, muscular system, and tendons and liga-ments. The last two are the foundation for strength. Without strong tendons and ligaments, it's like building a tall building without first digging deep into the ground.

Isometrics

Isometrics, sometimes referred to as dynamic ten-sion, is the process of using your body against itself. I'm using the word isometrics as an umbrella term. There are a lot of "iso's" out there: isometric, isotonic, isokinetic. For the sake of clarity, we'll just stick with isometrics. This requires even less equipment than calisthenics. Rest assured, if you're ever projected into outer space, you can still train. Place one hand below your chest, palm up. Then, with your other hand, push down against it. Hold for ten seconds, then switch to the other side. That's isometrics in a nutshell. There are isometric exercises for every part of the body. You can read more in depth about them in Charles Bronson's book, *Solitary Fitness*. Just keep in mind he has a colorful vocabulary and strong opinions. Isometrics is great for strength, but not so much for cardio since you aren't moving. Unless you add movement, you won't get very much in the range of motion, which I think is necessary in exercise. That's why I use isometrics for those hard-to-reach places, like my neck.

Yoga

You won't build any bodybuilder-type muscles in yoga, but you will build a strength and flexibility that few know. When you're in a difficult position, you breathe calmly. If you have problems under pressure, after some yoga, you'll find you're able to keep a calmer head. The reason more women do yoga than men is a cultural misunderstanding. Yes, women are more flexible, but men can certainly benefit from it as well. In fact, yoga was created for men, by men originally. It wasn't until much later that women were even allowed to do yoga when a young lady named Indra Devi was accepted as a student under Sri Krishnamacharya in 1937.[9] Yoga is more than just stretching, it creates balance and dexterity. But like most men, I had preconceived notions about yoga until it seriously kicked my butt— and it was a beginner's class! The most important strength is supple strength, and that's what you get from yoga. It is also somewhat intrusive because you twist and bend your body in weird ways. Maybe that's why men don't do it. There's also hot yoga, where you perform the exercises in a hot room. As if it wasn't tough enough!

Gymnastics

Gymnastics is in my opinion, what the pinnacle of fitness looks like. It's basically calisthenics on steroids. Think of the hardest things you can do with just your body to work out, and gymnastics makes it harder. Have you ever looked at a gymnast's biceps? They look like soft-balls. Not to mention they're doing the elite exercises that even people doing advanced calisthenics drool over: backflips, front flips, bridges, muscle-ups, etc. Learning gymnastics can take years. I list it here because I am in awe of it. But if you do learn and master it, you will have a level of fitness and flexibility that few realize.

Other types of training

There are many other types of training. Like I mentioned, do what works best for you. Yoga is great for building balance and flexibility. Weight training is great for building muscular strength. Experiment. Try different things. The truth is, they're all good for you, just in different ways. You just have to find the one that moves you towards what you want to accomplish.

CHAPTER FOURTEEN

DEVELOPING YOUR INNER TRAINER

When it comes to exercising on your own, you can push yourself to go farther or slow yourself down. You may not have a Mickey to yell at you, but you can be your own trainer when no one else is around.

Inner trainer?

What do I mean by inner trainer? Ever walk away from a workout early, only to feel disappointed in yourself because you didn't give it your all? Ever feel the desire to do a certain exercise that wasn't part of your routine that day but did it anyway? Ever not do an exercise you were supposed to do a particular day because you felt you shouldn't? That's your inner trainer. It's that whisper I spoke of that tells you what and what not to do in a workout, like a combination of your gut and intuition. Developing an inner trainer takes patience, it won't happen overnight. But with time, you'll be able to see what you need to do in your mind's eye. And it becomes clearer the more you work on it.

Listening to your body

When you're exercising, listen to your body: What do you need to do? What do you want to do? What is your body telling you? I used to be very strict with my workouts, I had a full regimen from the moment I stepped into the gym to the moment I stepped out. But it was so strict and structured, it suffocated any spontaneous flow of energy. In other words, if it was on the schedule, even if I didn't feel the need to do it, I did it anyway. This may sound very wishy-washy. *You mean do things you only feel like?* I'm not saying to avoid hard things, rather, feel in your body if you *should* be doing something. What is my body trying to tell me? A good example is me thinking I have to do more pullups. But that feeling not to do more is a tap on the shoulder. It means I'm missing something. And almost immediately when I don't do that extra set of pullups my brain was telling me I had to do, I remember that I was going to do muscle-ups. Instead of spinning my ego on the pullup bar, my body was trying to say it wanted to do something else, something more important. Get outside of your mind and into your body. That is where the vast ocean of wisdom is. Your body is trying to speak to you. Are you listening?

Mind's eye

When you're done exercising, think about what you did. When you're driving home, taking a shower, or eating afterwards, think. What did you do? What could you have done better? Where did you improve? What will you do tomorrow? What *won't* you do tomorrow? Think about your body, think about your workouts, see them in your mind. I've gotten to the point where I can see myself performing an exercise in my mind's eye. They say that when you picture yourself doing something in your head, the body fires the same muscles as if it's actually happening. High-performing athletes do this, they call it visualization. Again, it won't happen overnight, but if you're consistent and persistent, and make exercise a part of your life, you can develop this interesting phenomenon.

When to stop and when to keep going

You have to listen to your body when you exercise. If something doesn't feel right, stop. On the other hand, you have to know when to keep going. Like all things, it's a matter of balance. You have to be wise to the situation, especially when you are on your own. You are the athlete, the coach, and the doctor. You have to push yourself, but be mindful. No one will know better than you.

CHAPTER FIFTEEN

THINKING FOR BEST RESULTS?

I was debating whether or not to delete this chapter. I mean I get it, who needs more motivation? You know you're supposed to have a sharp mindset to work out. But I went through the chapter again and saw that it wasn't fluff. Nothing in this book is here to try and sell you something or make you like me. I want you to live healthy. And not just for a few weeks, but for a whole life to come.

Flexibility

We like to control things. We like to do what we want, how we want, and when we want. But sometimes things are outside of our control. Instead of trying to force the star piece into the square space, it is better to try and find more efficient ways of doing things. The person who suffers the most is the person who tries to control everything. Let's say you have a great exercise routine going. You wake up in the morning, go to work, come home and workout in the evening. You've been doing it for some time. But your boss is unaware of such trivialness and comes by your desk.

"Yeah... I'm going to need you to work overtime this week."

You have two choices: You can remain stubborn and still exercise after work, although it will be much later and you won't be getting as much sleep at night. Or you can just workout tomorrow morning instead. You go to bed when you get home and wake up early to exercise before work. Now you no longer need to kill yourself from being so stubborn and have a great new routine. Flexibility is the key to a healthy exercise routine because routines aren't set in stone. Life happens, it's just the ability to roll with the punches.

Adaptability

There may be times in your life you will have to sacrifice what you are doing for something entirely different. For me, it occurred while on deployment. I soon realized that working out for two to three hours after working fifteen was simply not realistic. I did it for a while, but sleep was catching up with me. Flexibility and adaptability are similar in that you let go of your stubborn ego and do the next best thing. Some might look at that as weak thinking but I look at it as the opposite. Being able to assess a situation and initiate the best form of action will not only help you to persevere but to move forward.

Because I was unable to lift weights for hours, and the five-by-five gyms were crowded with impatient sailors waiting for their turn on the machines, I had to find a way to exercise in half the time with double the results, and that's how I found calisthenics. But the moral of the story is not which workout is better, but which workout is most appropriate right now? Being adaptable doesn't mean you have to give up what you love, it means allowing it to transform and serve you, as opposed to you serving it. Don't be afraid to try new things because you may just discover exactly what you had been looking for.

Resoluteness

My father used to have a magnet on his refrigerator titled, "Everyone has an excuse." They ranged from the basic, *It started to rain* to the magnificent, *My psychic told me not to go out today*. Excuses are a great way to get out of something by coming up with anything. There were guys on deployment who'd say, *"Man, I can't work out, I just don't have the time!"* And when we got back they'd say, *"Man, I can't work out, there's just so much to do!"* It doesn't matter what kind of situation they're in, they always have an excuse. So don't be that guy (or gal). Be the person who says, "Man, it sucks I don't have much time, but damn it, I'm going to work out anyway." If you find yourself the kind of person who always has an excuse, try to reevaluate it. The more you say *yes* instead of *no* to your workouts the more you will be able to get things done. In fact, you'll go above and beyond to get your workouts in, even if it's just a small workout.

Chapter Sixteen

Motivation and Lack Thereof

Whether you're brand new to exercise or have been doing it for years, it is inevitable that you are going to get bored sooner or later. You'll lose focus and forget why you're working out. I like to step back from exercise time to time to look at the big picture and get a fresh perspective.

Boredom as a signal

Sometimes we get so immersed in our routines that we forget what we're even doing. You may have a day when you just don't have the gas or mental fortitude to exercise. I think those days are important because it's your body or mind's way of saying something's off. Boredom is a signal that something is wrong and needs your attention. It could be that you've burned yourself out, or you haven't given yourself a break in a long time. It could also just be that you're doing the same thing over and over and need a reminder of why you're even exercising.

Over-discipline chokes energy

I am all for discipline, but sometimes you can be too disciplined. Too disciplined, you say? I believe that the greatest workouts happen as a result of spontaneity, and spontaneity comes from creative energy. If you're constantly disciplined and know exactly what you're going to do and how you're going to do it, you're going to choke that energy and miss bigger things. Things that could better serve you. We think we know everything. We think we know what's good for us, but that's not always the case. In a previous chapter I talked about how listening to your gut can take you beyond your rational mind. Somedays you want to do something different. Listen to this, it may be your body trying to tell you something. Doing the same thing over and over again can get monotonous. Allowing some creative energy in the flow will spruce up your life and your workouts. Be spontaneous, do something different. It might just be the difference between the same old workout, and the best one of your life.

Learn and grow

On rare occasions I take a day off. A day off? Oh my gosh! Yes, blasphemy I know. I do this when I need a reset and I'm too close to my workouts. Why? Without forest fires, forests can't grow. I do this to expand my mind, so I use the time to catch up on my fitness reading. My mind is unsettled that I'm not working out so it latches onto something. I get my hands on an exercise book that interests me and learn something new. It's not enough to only exercise your body, you must also exercise your mind. Discover new exercises, better ways to eat, and even ways to improve what you're doing now. If you do this, I promise you will be eons ahead of someone who is only exercising their body.

Exercise is a relationship

There are countless ways to get back motivation and spruce up exercise again. An exercise and fitness routine is a relationship. It is a relationship between you and your body. And like any relationship, things can tend to wade off into the dull side after some time has passed. That doesn't mean you should just give up though. Add to your relationship, change things up, bring in some zest and pizzaz. Because the other choice you have is to do nothing. If you just keep at it, things will appear to you. Be creative, think outside the box, nobody said exercise had to be boring.

Here is a list of some things you could do to combat boredom in your exercise relationship:

- Try something new, like a new sport
- Take a day off, read, and learn something
- Change up your workouts, do something different
- Add a variation, like exercising outside
- Push yourself, do something harder

Think about the possible reasons why you're bored with your workouts. What is it you could be missing?

CHAPTER SEVENTEEN

OF SICKNESS AND HEALTH

Probably the worst thing to happen in the middle of an exercise routine is to get sick or injured. Everything stops. Everything. This is frustrating for someone who has worked hard to make the progress they have. A lot of thoughts will run through your head:

I was doing so well, now I'm going to lose everything!

How am I supposed to come back from this?

For some reason, when it rains it pours. One morning I woke up perfectly fine. I ate breakfast, did my morning routine, and took a shower. But when I got out, I started to feel weird. I got cold. I thought it was just a difference between temperatures. But when I got done getting dressed it hit me like a bus. I was out for a week. Unfortunately, we do get sick. It's just a part of being alive. If you exercise and eat well though, the times are fewer and far between.

Muscle memory

Muscle memory is the body's blueprint of things already achieved— like riding a bike. Muscle memory is a key component to exercise. Without it, every time you got sick or injured you'd have to start from scratch. Sometimes it feels like that, but you're further along than you think. Muscle memory helps you get back to where you were faster, and to remember the technicalities of how to perform specific exercises. But it's not just the muscles. It's also the ligaments, tendons, and bones that helped you do the work you were doing.

In the movie *Copland* starring Sylvester Stallone, Stallone takes on a character that is unlike all his others. We all know Stallone for his killer shape in action movies but for Copland he took on a different approach. His character is a sad and shy town cop. It wouldn't make sense for him to look like Rambo. He was, in a word, soft. So before filming, Stallone stopped all forms of exercise and threw his good eating habits out the window. He would go to his local diner every morning and eat five to seven huge pancakes smothered in syrup, followed by a glass of chocolate milk.

Stallone's body took on quite a transformation. He was bigger, but not necessarily badder. After filming was done, he put himself on a strict to-do list. He went to the gym and exercised like his life depended on it, and it probably did. He cut out the junk and started eating good foods again. Stallone was able to get back into shape in just a few weeks.

Stallone's is a special case because he has exercised for years. I'm not saying you can just slack off whenever you like and hope to rebound the next week. But it is helpful to know that if you ever get seriously sick or injured, it's not the end of the world, and you can certainly come back from it.

Healthy mind, healthy body

It may sound like New Age fluff, but people underestimate the power of the mind. When you think often about getting sick, you're going to get sick more often. Just like the placebos people take, I believe a lot of basic illnesses and allergies are just in our minds. People love to talk about their health problems. They talk about how their knees are bad and all the medications they're taking. It becomes a competition to see who's worse off.

Remember that story I told you about how I blew my foot out doing calf raises? Ironically, a similar thing happened to a guy I was working with. He went to medical and they told him he would have foot trouble for the rest of his life. I refused to listen to that, so I continued to walk on the foot, believing it would heal itself. And you know what? It did. Not only did it heal itself, but it got stronger than my other foot. Most people think that the body comes first and the mind comes second, but it's actually the other way around. The mind comes first and the body comes second. If you believe you are sick and you won't get better, your chances of staying sick longer and not getting well are much higher. I'm not saying this as a magical remedy to severe cases, you should not just forgo necessary medical treatment where it is vital. But it is important to know that your mind plays a critical role in your health. In fact, it plays the most critical role.

If you're going to be healthy, it's not enough to only exercise and eat right, you need to make health your mindset. When you talk to people, choose your words wisely. Even if our thoughts really did not become things, at the very least they can create a lot of unnecessary worry.

Chapter Eighteen

Divvying up the Body

Dividing the body up into different parts is important because we want to make sure that everything is getting exercised respectively. The key to a good exercise routine is organization. The same goes for a healthy life. When you're sloppy and disorganized your chances of staying healthy are few and far between. Here we are going to divide up the different parts of the body that are going to be exercised. The most important thing we need is balance.

Dividing the body into workout sessions

These are the four main sections of the body that need to be exercised. There should be balance in your body. You don't want to be constantly pulling and forget about pushing. We want everything worked respectively.

1. Push
2. Pull
3. Legs
4. Lower back
5. Abs

Push: <u>Pushups</u>. If you can't do regular pushups, you can do knee pushups. If you can't do knee pushups, you can do wall pushups, an even simpler form of exercise. Pushups work the chest and are a favorite of Batman. I would recommend calisthenics (body exercises) to any new beginner in exercise. This is because you can adjust the difficulty in a plethora of ways, but more importantly because it builds strong tendons and ligaments. That way if you ever do decide to go to the bench-press, you'll have a solid foundation.

Pull: I would love to recommend pull-ups to you, but that may be a little too advanced. In the mean-time there is the <u>lateral pull-down machine</u>. You can find one in any gym. It has a bench and a horizontal bar hanging at the top. You pull the bar down to your chest. The machine is connected to weights on the side, which can be adjusted accordingly. This works your upper back muscles. It's like a seated pull-up. One of my favorite exercises in general.

Legs: While running could be considered legs, I'm going to keep it separate as a form of cardio. For legs, I'm going to go with the tried and true <u>squat</u>. Squats are better than any leg exercise, and you don't need a squat rack if you're just beginning. Just down, and up. If you have knee problems, consult with a doctor first, or just stick with cardio, such as walking or light jogging. The squat is fantastic because it works all the leg muscles in unison (quadriceps, hamstrings, calves, feet, toes), as opposed to a lot of other leg machines that isolate the muscles.

Lower back: <u>The bridge</u>. I will go into more depth with the bridge in the next chapter. But for now, let's just cover the basics. The bridge is like a backwards pushup. You lie on your back, put your hands up and over your head and onto the floor behind you. Then you push up. Again, as with all exercises and workouts in this book, especially ones you may be unfamiliar with, consult a doctor before you perform any of them. This is a simple version of the bridge, and one of the most important, and yet unheard of, exercises. In the next chapter I will explain why it is important, and its relationship with the abs.

Abs: For the abdominals we're going to go with the simple <u>sit-up</u>. For the sit-up it's good to have something holding your feet down. If you don't have someone to do it, try finding something you can place them under, such as a bed or a dresser for support. Obviously you can do it without support, but it will be a little more difficult. I suggest support if you are relatively new, so as to not put too much pressure on the lower back.

Balance

Your body needs to be balanced—everything needs to be exercised respectively. If you do too much of one thing it's going to create an imbalance between parts of the body. And a body that works in harmony is a dangerous thing. We'll have to put you in a cage, kid.

Chapter Nineteen

Overlooked and Often Misused Parts of the Body

There are parts of the body that don't get the attention they deserve. This leads to pain, stiffness, and imbalance. I think we forget that the body is a machine, with all the parts working in unison.

Muscles have relationships

Most muscle groups have a sister/brother relationship: the biceps and triceps, the quadriceps and hamstrings, the abdominals and lower back. When you exercise one, you can't neglect the other. This may sound like common sense, but for some people, they may not exercise a particular muscle group because they're more interested in another (the biceps over the triceps) or they don't understand the relationship (the front abs and the lower back). To have a singularly worked body, every muscle group needs to be taken into account, and the relationships between muscles need to be understood.

Lower-back

Not only is the lower back the most overlooked part of the body, it's also the most important when it comes to good posture and getting rid of back pain. As people get stronger, they tend to load the abs with heavier weight, while simultaneously neglecting (or abusing) the lower back. This creates a crater between two opposing muscle groups: the front abs and the lower back (spinal erectors).

The hyperextension is an exercise where you stand on a platform and move your body forward to a ninety-degree angle. The problem with this is it severely tightens the lower back. While this can be good for other parts of the body, it's not good for the spinal erectors because instead of needing tightened, they need to be stretched and massaged. That's how they get stronger. Strength isn't just about how much weight you can lift but how flexible the muscles are. The spinal erectors, or lower back muscles, need to be massaged. Not in the sense that someone should stand on them (though that does sound nice) but in the sense that the movements which are performed open up and stretch them.

The relationship between the lower back and abs

Overworking the abs strains the lower back. Imagine putting a book bag on in front of you and you start putting rocks in the bag. It sucks. The lower back tries to compensate for the load but doesn't have the means to support itself, it becomes strained. This is what happens when you overwork the abs and neglect the lower back. When the abs are too tight, and the lower back is too weak, you're pulled forward and slouch. We exercise our abs so that we can have a six-pack. But we neglect the other muscles that work with them and this causes major problems.

The Bridge

I watched this monk training in an anime. There were some quick scene changes. First, he was doing pushups. Then he was doing sit-ups. And then he was doing what I could only describe as backwards push-ups. It was supposed to be funny. I laughed. But that's kind of what a bridge is. It's an exercise that works your spinal erectors— one of the most important exercises you may never have heard of. Lie on your back, put your hands on the floor overhead. Push your body up. That's a beginner's bridge. If you want to go more in-depth, there are plenty of videos on YouTube. But DO NOT try to do a full, stand-to-floor bridge until you've mastered the easier bridge exercises.

Posture

In Guam, a friend of mine pointed out something I never noticed before, he said I slouched. A lot of people don't notice that they do, but fixing it is easy. He told me to just pull my chest up like there was an invisible string attached to the top of my head. Posture isn't just a way of looking better when you walk, it helps your back, in particular the spinal erectors. You don't have to puff your chest out like you want to fight somebody, but noticing that you slouch and straightening your back can make a world of difference, even though it's a simple thing.

Hamstrings

Hamstrings are tricky to isolate and I believe there is a good reason for this: they're not meant to be isolated. When they are, it causes another imbalance between two major muscle groups: the quadriceps and the hamstrings. If you've ever taken martial arts, you know just how tight the hamstrings are. This is what I mean when I say stretching is strengthening. Imagine a rubber band.

If it is too thin, it snaps. If it's too thick, it's not flexible. But if it's medium taut, it's both strong and flexible; the Goldilocks's zone. Everything in the Universe is balance, the hamstrings are no exception. If you want strong and flexible hamstrings, stay away from machines that isolate them, and work them conjunctively with the quadriceps. That's where squats come in. You can't do a squat without both muscle groups working simultaneously. And don't forget to stretch, the hamstrings are stronger the more flexible they are. Flexibility creates durability.

CHAPTER TWENTY

BEGINNING EXERCISE

If you're reading this, you may be new to exercise, so I want you to understand some important things before you do a single push up. And even if you aren't new, it's good to have a refresher. If you decide to take the gym route (or even if you work out at home) and aren't already preoccupied by another means of exercising, i.e., swimming, yoga, etc., this chapter can help you.

Before

There's nothing worse than getting hurt when you could've prevented it. But warming up and stretching appear to be optional anymore; a lot of people don't seem to do it. But unless you want to end up in a cast, I suggest starting the right way.

Stretching: Imagine a piece of frozen taffy. Take a hammer to it and it smashes to pieces. Warm up that same taffy and the hammer just leaves an imprint. Stretching gets the muscles loose and ready for the work to come.

Warming Up: Some people say stretching is part of the warmup. For the sake of clarity though, we'll keep the two separate. Stretching opens up the muscles and joints. Warming up gets your heart pumping. Some people like to do light cardio before they exercise. Others like to wear heavy clothing. Either way is fine, they both do the same thing— get you warmed up.

Sets and reps

What is a set? And what is a rep for that matter?

The best way I have come to define them is:

Rep: The number of times a movement is performed in an exercise.

Set: The number of times an exercise is performed in a workout.

For example: I did 4 sets of push-ups. Each set had 10 reps. So, I did a total of 40 push-ups.

Warm-up sets: Before you get to your harder exercises, you have to get your muscles warmed up first. The point of warm-up sets is to get the muscles ready for your working sets.

<u>Working sets</u>: These are the hard sets of your workout. The ones you prepared for in your warm-up sets.

Here's an example:

(1) *Warm-up set*: Push-ups, 5 Reps (1 set)

(1) *Warm-up set*: Push-ups, 5 Reps

(1) <u>Working set</u>: Push-ups, 10 Reps

(1) <u>Working set</u>: Push-ups, 15 Reps

Introductory workouts

The workouts I am about to share with you are introductory. While anyone can do them, they're geared more specifically to those who are newer to exercise. These are to be used as a guide map to get you comfortable with working out. When you get more proficient, you can advance to more strenuous workouts.

Remember the chapter, *Divvying up the Body*? Here we're going to put those divisions to good use.

1. Full- Body Workout:

A full- body workout is just that, full- body. Here you're going to exercise every muscle group three times a week. Twice if you feel less confident, and so on. For the sake of clarity, I'm going to make the schedule as if we are exercising three times a week.

Monday: Push, Pull, Legs, Abs, Lower back

Tuesday: Off, or Light Cardio (brisk walking, jogging, swimming, biking, etc.)

Wednesday: Push, Pull, Legs, Abs, Lower back

Thursday: Off, or Light Cardio (brisk walking, jogging, swimming, biking, etc.)

Friday: Push, Pull, Legs, Abs, Lower back

Saturday: Off, or Light Cardio (brisk walking, jogging, swimming, biking, etc.)

Sunday: Off.

2. Split- Body Workout:

The split-body workout is just as it sounds: you split the body over the course of the week. It's a little more advanced, and you can get more work done in the week because now you are focusing more time on fewer muscle groups each day. You can give them more love.

Monday: Push, Pull, Legs.

Tuesday: Abs, Lower back.

Wednesday: Off, or Light Cardio.

Thursday: Push, Pull, Legs.

Friday: Abs, Lower back.

Saturday: Off, or Light Cardio.

Sunday: Off.

You can see that I usually have Sunday off. That's just a personal preference and you don't have to adhere to it. These are just a couple of simple workouts anyone can do, and are particularly geared towards beginners. They're meant to be simple, yet effective. And as I mentioned, they can be adjusted to the individual's needs to be made either harder or easier.

Chapter Twenty-one

Expanding Your Fitness Universe

There are many paths in fitness. If you're tired of doing the same old thing, or if you're in a rut, you may want to see what else is out there. It's a great way to challenge yourself, open your mind, and be humbled. While this may seem very similar to the chapter *Different Types of Training*, this is less specific to different kinds of exercise, i.e., weightlifting, calisthenics, etc., and more specific to ways you can use your body, be that sports or aerobic activity.

Swimming

If I was stranded on an island and had to choose one form of exercise for the rest of my life, I would choose swimming. Not only because it's probably the best workout you can do, but also because I'd be able to swim off the island. But then again, I might swim back. Swimming is everything you could want rolled into one: cardio, stretching, muscle work, and meditation. You use your body against the water's resistance, so you don't have to worry about overdoing it. That's why people still swim in their old age, and parents bring their babies to swim too. It keeps your heart healthy and is easy on the bones. I love swimming, but I know how intimidating the water can be, especially if you weren't brought up learning how to swim. Go slow, learn basic movements and get comfortable in the water. That's the most important thing I can tell you. Become a fish. And even if all you do is doggy paddle, at least you're in the water. An excellent introductory course to swimming is Terry Laughlin's book *Total Immersion*. He shows you how swimming can be made effortless and enjoyable, as opposed to simply pushing harder in the water.

Tennis

When we stopped in Guam, I had a chance to play tennis with a buddy of mine, the one who told me I slouched. Our hotel had a court and we were bored. So we thought it would be a fun idea to hit the ball back and forth. But it's no joke! Tennis has you running all over the place like a madman. And you have to be concentrated on the ball at all times. I challenge you to give it a try. They make it look easy on TV.

Just a tip: Alternate the sides of your body. Some coaches make their players use only their good side, but it's better to be balanced. If you're only good on one side and get hurt, that's it. But if you better your weak side, your good side will improve also.

Self-defense

Learning self-defense is a noble undertaking. Being fit is one thing, but using your body to protect others is another. I've taken a few Tai Kwon Do classes and my hips never got such a beating. But I kept at it, and within a few days, I could do the movements better. If you decide to do self-defense, research the different kinds. See what's available near you, though I've heard of people driving very far because they wanted a specific style or instructor. You'll find strength, flexibility, and balance you never knew. Young or old, it's a great thing to consider. Before you start handing over wads of cash though, ask if you can take some free classes. Finding the right teacher is like finding a pair of jeans that fit just right.

Boxing

Boxing is one heck of a sport. You'll get stamina,

speed, and strength. But the hardest thing about boxing is getting punched. Once you get over that though, you can go a long way. Boxing is very physical, but it's still more mental. If you want to just train, that's fine. It's a good workout. But getting in the ring is harder than any boxing workout you can perform. It tests you and puts you in the fire. Most people do not like getting punched, and for good reason. But if you find that you still want to do it, even after getting punched in the face, then maybe it's for you. You'll reap a lot of rewards. Just use your boxing skills for good, and only in the ring.

Challenge yourself

These are just a few of the many different kinds of sports and ways you can use your fitness. Find something that makes you grow. Find what speaks to you. And it doesn't have to be expensive. Just because something costs a lot doesn't mean it's worth your time. The best things in life are free, like playing frisbee in the park!

Chapter Twenty-two

Parting Wisdom

What do we do now? As important as it is to have a destination in mind, it's more important to take the first step. Anything you do for the first time is going to be challenging. It does get easier though. Hopefully not your workouts, but being healthy.

Temple

Picture the Pyramids of Egypt. All conspiracy theories aside, they were built to house the dead pharaohs. So as amazing as they are, they weren't built to just be looked at. They were built for a purpose, and to house something important.

Your body also houses something important. You have a heart that pumps blood throughout your body and you have a brain that stores massive amounts of information. Your body is made up of trillions of cells. You have hands and fingers and opposable thumbs. You have lungs that breathe air. You have kidneys that protect your body from toxins and even eyebrows that keep sweat out of your eyes. Your body does so much for you, and it houses so many treasures. Do you take care of the gifts you've been given?

Role models

Some people enjoy looking at pictures of physically fit people they admire. Arnold Schwarzenegger did this. Even though this can help, it's not necessary. You'll never look exactly like someone else because we're all built differently. We all have noses but they all look different. When you strive to look exactly like someone else, it becomes obsessive. But it doesn't hurt to have someone you look up to. It's only when it gets out of hand that it becomes a problem. I was raised on the Rocky films, and I'll always marvel at Stallone's physique, but I don't try to emulate him anymore. I develop the body I have, in the way that I do. And to me, that's more important than trying to copy someone else.

Never stop learning

You don't have to be a fitness buff to learn more about exercise. Pick up books. Read. Your body and mind work together. Without one, the other can't be the best it can be. Books are great, but if something doesn't sit right with you, question it. Don't just blindly follow. I've heard it said that the best religion is the one that you make for yourself. Exercise is the same way. If you don't believe in what you're doing, then what's the point of doing it at all?

Your weak points

We like to work on our strengths. If we have strong legs, we make them the focus of our workouts. If we have weak arms, we complain that mother nature wasn't kind to us. But if you want to get better, don't just focus on what you're good at, work on what you're not. For me, I've always had trouble running. My endurance was poop. But I ran and I ran, and eventually it sucked less and less. When you work on your weak points, you balance yourself out. There's a chasm between your strengths and your weaknesses. You can narrow the bridge.

One at a time

Exercise can be overwhelming. If all you're ever thinking about is what needs to get done next, you'll never stick with what you're doing now. But if you learn to be mindful, you can take it one step at a time. Approach every workout as its own being—the workout you are doing today is the only one that exists—not yesterdays, not tomorrows. Because for some people, unfortunately, tomorrow never comes. One workout at a time, one exercise at a time, one set at a time, one rep at a time. The smaller you can make each bite, the better you can digest what you're doing.

Simple

A good workout doesn't have to be complicated. In fact, the best ones aren't. If you strip everything down to its basics, you won't need to use half your energy to think about what needs to be done. The moment you forget the reason why you're working out, stand back. Reevaluate. Chop off the complicated, and get back into it. Think and be aware. "Do I need to be doing this?" "What is the point of me doing this?" "How is this making me better?"

It doesn't have to be expensive

If you think that you have to jump into exercise with fancy shoes, notebooks that measure micro/macronutrients, and three hundred dollar workout clothes, you'll hype yourself up and come crashing down. Keep it simple. You don't need fancy or expensive. Grab what you have and go from there.

Better than nothing

Something is always better than nothing. I don't care what it is— a few pushups, a walk around the park, anything. Often, doing just a little leads to doing more. But even if that's not the case, that's okay. The important thing is to do something. Too tired to work out? Crank out a few push-ups. Need to go to the store? Put on your walking shoes.

A tapestry

I was listening to the radio one day and the host was talking about how Americans were polled on how long they eat healthy during the week until they falter. They said that most had the best intentions on Monday, but by Wednesday, they were eating pizza and wings. There is a simple reason for this, one that has kept me in good shape for years: Eating healthy alone is not going to keep you fit. If you focus only on a healthy diet, you're missing the other half of the equation, which is to exercise. It's a dance of dragons, and the two keep each other accountable. You know that you have to exercise (or already have) and if you eat crappy, you waste (or wasted) your workout. This has also kept me from cigarettes and alcohol. Instead of nicotine, exercise kills my stress. And alcohol dehydrates me and hurts my muscles. It's all sewn together in one large tapestry.

Balance

There is an idea out there that too much exercise can be bad for you. They say that when you run excessively, it builds up scar tissue over the heart. I can't say if this is true, people run marathons and do incredible things with their bodies. But I have heard of people "fit as a fiddle" drop dead. Why? If there is any truth to this, I think it comes down to balance. It is a lot of strain on the body to be operating at one hundred percent, one hundred percent of the time. Can it do it? Yes. People push the body in remarkable ways. But they do it in increments, or for special occasions during specific parts of their lives. Give your body some rest, allow it to recover. Exercise to better yourself. Obsession has its place, but keep in mind that the ego is a never satiated black hole. The ego will never be satisfied, but the self can be.

Like a car

Your body is like a car. It needs to be maintained. When it is not looked after, it breaks down. When it's not given proper fuel, it runs out of gas. When it is not taken care of, it rusts and falls apart.

Soap and shampoo

I used to shower every day, using plenty of body wash, shampoo, and hair conditioner. But too much soap and shampoo is not good for your hair and skin. Your body has natural oils that you strip every time you use them. I'm not saying you should never use these products, rather, use them sparingly.

Using water sparingly

I shower a few times a week, occasionally using soap. Eww, yuck! Yeah, I know. But you don't stink like everyone says you will. Honestly, water is enough on its own most of the time. That alone dries out your hair and skin. This doesn't just help my body but also saves money on water and soap. More importantly, it saves hundreds of gallons of otherwise wasted water. Water is a luxury here in the U.S. There are countries where people walk miles just to get water. Like my friend once said, "You know you live in a rich country when, even in a crappy place, you can find a water fountain."

Your kids involved

If you have kids, get them involved in sports—especially at an early age. It will help them grow mentally, physically, and socially. The ability to make friends can't be exaggerated either. I'm sure you have heard it before but it bears repeating that sports help kids learn values and function well in social situations. It's a great microcosm for the bigger world. And it's imperative to be supportive. Let your kid choose what they like, but when they do, be there for them. If they want to change sports, ask them why. But make sure it's not because of an embarrassment or a misunderstanding.

Bonus Chapter I

Making Exercise a Part of Your Life

Exercising can be difficult but it doesn't have to be a chore. I challenge you to enjoy your workouts. Don't stress out about them during the day. Don't think to yourself, "Oh no, I have to work out later!" Just go about your day, and when it's time to exercise, exercise. If it becomes a tedious task, then you'll stop doing it and never want to do it again. It hasn't always been easy for me to work out. When I was younger, I used to get sick to my stomach at the thought of it. But over time I got better and then it became a part of my life. Today I cannot not exercise.

Why exercise?

We're all growing older. Unless someone discovers the fountain of youth, that's just how it is. So why not keep yourself feeling younger longer? Of course, I'm not suggesting you spend three hours in the gym every day. It's like the paradox, "You work out to live longer but you spend half your life in the gym." For me, exercise is meditation; when I can stop thinking about the troubles of my day and just work out. It's not something I do to punish myself, rather something I do to better myself. Not just physically, but mentally as well.

An unnecessary inconvenience

Fitness is optional, that's why we're so out of shape. Centuries ago, humans didn't have a choice but to be physical. Whether fighting for their dinner or running for their lives, they had to move. Today we don't. We don't have to hunt or fish. That's someone else's job. There are no mobs of animals chasing us, and we don't have to worry about being thrown into a cage with another person and fighting to the death. Rome got complacent too; the rich immersed themselves in pleasure. They relished their lifestyle of sex, wine and parties, that's why it fell. Fitness may be optional today but that doesn't mean it's any less important.

Do it for them

Make the decision for you but also for the important people in your life. If you have kids, do it for them. Be a role model for fitness. Help them make healthy choices. They don't need to be like those Russian weightlifting kids, but they'll be much more willing to eat their vegetables if they see mom or dad doing it. If you have kids, you know they mimic everything you do. When I was little, my dad used to slurp his coffee. I didn't know he was doing it because it was hot, but I mimicked him all the same with my cold juice. Never underestimate the power of a child's perception.

Bonus Chapter II

Cold Showers

I remember a guy I worked with telling me about Bond showers; showers that start hot and end cold. The idea is you open your pores, clear them out, and close them back up. I wish someone had told me about cold showers years ago. It baffles me that we're not told regularly about the benefits.

Shiver me timbers!

For me, I was looking for a way to build mental toughness, and in the process found how good cold showers are for you. They do build up mental tenacity, but there's more to them than just the psychological aspect. There are a lot of health benefits to cold showers too: better blood circulation, healthier hair, and clearer skin. And so the opposite is true of hot showers. I know, they feel good, especially in the morning. But they decrease fertility, cause a multitude of skin problems, and even lower sperm count.[10] Check out this really cool article on cold showers by The Art of Manliness.[11]

Building up to

Most people say the best way to take a cold shower is to take a cold shower. While that certainly is the fastest approach, I recommend doing it a little differently. When I was younger, I had to take a lot of cold showers. Our hot water ran off of a gas tank and we couldn't always fill it up. When that happened, I had to make a choice: take a cold shower, or go to school smelling like a fish (or so I thought.) What was worse, our shower was in the basement, which was already cold, especially in the winter. The bathroom upstairs only had a tub, and I never liked baths. To top it off, there was a window in the basement people always forgot to close. So it's the middle of winter, no hot water, and the window's open. I should've been nominated for the Polar Bear Club. When I got out, it would take me a few minutes to remember who I was and what I was doing in the basement.

Don't do that if you can avoid it. Instead, work up to cold showers. At the end of your normal shower, dial back the heat a little, enough you can take. As you take more showers, make them a little colder.

Pretty soon, you'll be taking showers others would run far and fast from. It's up to you if you want to take them straight, or start hot and end cold (Bond shower.) Straight cold showers are great after a workout, it's like jumping into a swimming pool. Back in the day, unless you were lucky enough to find a hot spring, people didn't have access to automated hot water. Cold is the way nature intended.

Surrender

There's nothing more nerve-wracking than standing outside your shower, butt naked, already shivering from the prospect of immersing yourself in cold water. How do you not freak out? You can take a cold shower squealing like a little piggy, but it will only add to the unpleasantries. Embrace the cold, don't fight it. When you exaggerate it, you make it more difficult than it needs to be. Just hop in, let the water run over you, and surrender. If you rush and fumble around, you'll knock things over and bang your elbow against the wall. Be efficient. This helps outside the shower too: staying calm and being able to focus in uncomfortable situations. All of this is obviously easier said than done. It will take time, and it will take practice. But if you master the art of the cold shower, it will be an invaluable tool in your health and wellness toolkit.

GYM ETIQUETTE

Not all of us will be going to the gym. Some of us might enjoy working out in our rooms, the park, or on a tree. But if you do find yourself surrounded by other people exercising, here are some universal rules you should be aware of.

1. <u>Wipe it down</u>: When you're done running on the treadmill or sitting on a machine, get a spray and towel, and wipe it down. Gyms are dirty enough. Plus, you don't want somebody slipping and hurting themselves on your sweat.
2. <u>Don't make conversation</u>: Most people go to the gym to, you guessed it, workout. Don't bother someone by talking sports or your new favorite hipster band. Asking a quick question is okay. Discussing current affairs is not.
3. <u>Turn your music *down*</u>: Not everyone likes the same music you do. I know, surprising right? And nobody wants to hear you burp out every other line of your song. Get a pair of headphones that are noise cancelling, or at least keep the volume below an eardrum splitting decibel.

4. <u>Don't grunt</u>: The gym isn't a zoo. If you can't exercise without screaming, then maybe workout outside. No one wants to hear you exaggerate that ten-pound weight you're lifting.

5. <u>Be mindful</u>: Other people in the gym want to work out too. If you're going to be somewhere for a while (squat rack) and feel a burning sensation on the back of your neck, ask that person if they'd like to take turns. On the other hand, if you're just texting or talking, you should know that we're trying to leave too.

6. <u>Put the weights *back*</u>! I can't tell you how many times I've walked to the dumbbell rack and can't find a weight's twin. Did somebody take just *one* dumbbell? After I look everywhere, I find it tucked behind a machine, in the corner of the gym. Sometimes they're gone completely. Don't be a blue falcon. And if they're lying on the floor, ask. People don't like when you steal their weights.

7. <u>Don't hoard: </u>There are people who like to collect weights. Maybe you've seen them; they have two twenties, two thirties, and a barbell. Put the weights back. If the weight you're hoping to use disappears, improvise. It won't kill you to alternate five or ten pounds.

Thank you for taking the time to read my book. I hope it has helped you and will continue to be a source of wisdom and inspiration for the rest of your healthy life. I am always interested in making the book better, so if you have any questions, please email me at: davidleasure@trulyhealthynow.com

Thank you.

BIBLIOGRAPHY

These are my teachers. They kept me company when I was alone and revolutionized how I thought about health and fitness. Without them this book doesn't exist. I'm not saying they have to be your teachers, but it might help to find your own. Read books, learn often. Find who speaks to you.

- Wade, Paul. *Convict Conditioning: How to Bust Free of All Weakness Using the Lost Secrets of Supreme Survival Strength.* Little Canada, MN: Dragon Door Publications, 2018.

This book is the foundation of my fitness. Though I started with Convict Conditioning 2, this first book lays the foundation for advanced calisthenics.

- Wade, Paul. *Convict Conditioning 2: Advanced Prison Training Tactics for Muscle Gain, Fat Loss, and Bulletproof Joints.* Little Canada, MN: Dragon Door Publications, 2018.

CC2 goes into greater detail than the first one. It's not necessary for a beginner who is interested in calisthenics, but it is always there if you find yourself moving past what is in the first one. It's more detail-oriented.

- Bronson, Charles, and Stephen Richards. *Solitary Fitness*. London: John Blake, 2007.

The book that started it all for me. I was given this book at a low point in my life. I felt connected to Bronson and his situation because ours felt similar. This book, however, is not for those with virgin ears—Bronson doesn't sugarcoat his words or how he feels about the current physical state of society.

- Stallone, Sylvester, and David Hochman. *Sly Moves: My Proven Program to Lose Weight, Build Strength, Gain Will Power, and Live Your Dream*. New York: Harper Collins, 2005.

Like I mentioned in the beginning of the book, I grew up on the Rocky films. And seeing as Stallone (as I am writing this) is in his seventies and in better physical shape than most twenty-year-old's, it would be smart to hear what he has to say. The book is simple, to the point, and dare I say it, motivational. A book that I always return to.

- Lauren, Mark, and Joshua Clark. *You Are Your Own Gym: The Bible of Bodyweight Exercises*. New York, NY: Ballantine Books, 2011.

This is an interesting book. Mark Lauren was a special ops guy (though he never comes out directly to say which.) He came to enlightenment about simple fitness, using your own body and things you have around you. It's a good read, and there are plenty of things to pick up from it.

- Kubik, Brooks D. *Dinosaur Bodyweight Training.* Louisville, KY: Brooks Kubik Enterprises, 2011.

More of an advanced book, but this is where I learned of the *mind/muscle* link.

- Laughlin, Terry, and John Delves. *Total Immersion: The Revolutionary Way to Swim Better, Faster, and Easier.* New York, NY: Fireside, 2004.

I came across this book when I was learning how to swim. It's an excellent resource for those wanting to find a more enjoyable way to learn swimming, instead of just pushing harder in the water. Terry Laughlin developed a whole science behind it, believing there was an easier way to swim, going against years of old-fashioned thinking from traditional swim coaches.

- Stanislavsky, Konstantin. *An Actor Prepares.* Routledge, 1989.

You can always find wisdom in no matter what you read.

REFERENCES

[1] "The Winter Warlock." Christmas Specials Wiki. Accessed January 13, 2022. https://christmas-specials.fandom.com/wiki/The_Winter_Warlock.

[2] Gay, Abbigail. "You Are Taller in the Morning Than You Are at Night." AREUFIT Health Services. August 20, 2020. https://www.areufithealthservices.com/you-are-taller-in-the-morning-than-you-are-at-night/.

[3] Silver, Natalie. "Why Does My Weight Fluctuate?" Healthline. July 31, 2018. Accessed October 14, 2018. https://www.healthline.com/health/weight-fluctuation.

[4] Howe, Russ. "How Sylvester Stallone Has Adapted His Training Over The Years." Russ Howe PTI. Accessed October 30, 2018. https://russhowepti.com/how-sylvester-stallone-has-adapted-his-training-over-the-years/.

[5] Yetman, Daniel. "Endurance Vs. Stamina: Differences and Tips to Improve Both." Healthline.

June 12, 2020. Accessed January 02, 2022. https://www.healthline.com/health/exercise-fitness/endurance-vs-stamina.

[6] Water Science School. "The Water in You: Water and the Human Body Completed." U.S. Geological Survey. May 22, 2019. Accessed October 27, 2018. https://www.usgs.gov/special-topics/water-science-school/science/water-you-water-and-human-body.

[7] Chandler, Adam. "Fake News Story: 'Bodybuilder Shot a 20 -Year-Old Guy for Asking Him 'Do You Even Lift?'." Adam Chandler's Blog. July 16, 2013. https://adamchandler.me/blog/2013/07/16/fake-news-story-bodybuilder-shot-a-20-year-old-guy-for-asking-him-do-you-even-lift/.

[8] "Supplements SEALgrinderPT Recommends and Uses." SEALgrinderPT. March 22, 2020. Accessed January 02, 2022. https://sealgrinderpt.com/supplements/.

[9] Caplan, Heather. "The Irony of Our Modern Female-Dominated Yoga." Spright. August 13, 2015. Accessed October 27, 2018. https://web.archive.org/web/20200724163948/http://archive.spright.com:80/exercises/history-of-women-practicing-yoga.

[10] Western, Dan. "7 Reasons to Stop Taking Hot Showers Every Morning." Wealthy Gorilla. Accessed January 11, 2017. https://wealthygorilla.com/5-reasons-stop-taking-hot-showers/.

[11] McKay, Brett & Kate. "The James Bond Shower: A Shot of Cold Water for Health and Vitality." The Art of Manliness. September 17, 2019. Accessed October 27, 2018. https://www.artofmanliness.com/articles/the-james-bond-shower-a-shot-of-cold-water-for-health-and-vitality/.

ACKNOWLEDGEMENTS

Thank you to the Navy and everyone who gave me a hard time. Without you, the insights would never have occurred, and this book would never have been written. Thank you to everyone who helped with editing this book, including my sister who was a big help.

ABOUT THE AUTHOR

David joined the Navy right out of high school. He was stationed in Japan and spent four years attached to a carrier. Even though it wasn't all sunshine and daisies, it gave him the lessons he needed to learn about health, fitness, and even spirituality.